The book that's helping thousands who are ill,
and thousands who want to stay well.

# ANATOMY OF AN ILLNESS

As perceived by the patient
Norman Cousins
Reflections on Healing and Regeneration

"Intriguing . . . He touches on such large topics as creativity, longevity and pain, and raises timely questions about holistic vs. traditional medicine, treating patients vs. treating diseases."

—*Newsweek*

"Cousins' reflections generated by his extraordinary triumph over a crippling illness are as inspiring as they are informed, as well stated as they are carefully conceived . . . It will be of great interest to those whose lives are touched by illness, and all who desire to increase their understanding and appreciation of being well."

—*Library Journal*

"His book will bring hope to many who need it and perhaps open up a new field for medical research."
—*John Barkham Reviews*

D0029400

# Anatomy of an Illness as Perceived by the Patient

REFLECTIONS ON HEALING AND REGENERATION

*by*

## NORMAN COUSINS

*Introduction by*

## RENÉ DUBOS

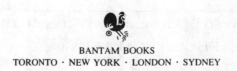

BANTAM BOOKS
TORONTO · NEW YORK · LONDON · SYDNEY

ANATOMY OF AN ILLNESS AS PERCEIVED BY THE PATIENT
*A Bantam Book / published by arrangement with*
*W. W. Norton & Co., Inc.*

*PRINTING HISTORY*
*Norton edition published September 1979*
*13 printings through September 1980*
*A Book-of-the-Month Club Special Spring Selection 1980*
*A Selection of Book Digest January 1980*
*Serialized in* EVENT MAGAZINE, *Summer 1980;* FAMILY CIRCLE,
*June 1980;* HEALTH QUARTERLY, OVATION MAGAZINE, *and*
UNITED FEATURES SYNDICATE
*Bantam edition / March 1981*
*6 printings through May 1985*

ISBN 0-553-01491-9

*Published simultaneously in the United States and Canada*

PRINTED IN THE UNITED STATES OF AMERICA
DH      15  14  13  12  11  10

For my brother Robert and
my sisters Sophie and Jeanne.

# CONTENTS

# ANATOMY OF AN ILLNESS
## AS PERCEIVED BY THE PATIENT

# INTRODUCTION

## by René Dubos

T he basic theme of this book is that every person must accept a certain measure of responsibility for his or her own recovery from disease or disability. This notion of patient responsibility is not new, of course, but the general philosophy behind the notion has seldom been stated better than in this book. Though the author is a layman, his ideas have achieved wide acceptance by the medical profession. His perceptions about the nature of stress and about the ability of the human mind to mobilize the body's capacity to combat illness are in accord with important findings at leading medical research centers.

It is inevitable, of course, that any book about the

healing phenomenon will lead to considerations of longevity. To be sure, this book is as much concerned with the quality of life as it is with the prolongation of life. Nevertheless, this dual emphasis of this volume fits in with one of the significant trends in modern society, namely, the general increase of life expectancy into the seventies and eighties. Indeed, according to a Social Security Administration report, there were 10,700 centenarians across the nation in 1976. The percentage of centenarians to total population is probably much the same in several other countries.

Admittedly, it is often difficult to prove the exact age of very old persons because records of their birthdates tend to be inexact or lacking altogether. In the United States, for example, the fully authenticated number of real centenarians may not reach ten thousand. Yet there are enough well-documented cases of very old people to prove that longevity can be achieved under many different climatic and social conditions.

In 1635, an Englishman, Thomas Parr, was summoned to London by Charles I because it had been reported to the king that church records and other circumstantial evidence showed "Old Parr"—as he was affectionately called—to be 152 years old. Old Parr was dined and wined, but died shortly thereafter, while still in London. An autopsy was performed by none other than William Harvey, who pronounced Parr's organs to be quite sound, "as healthy as the day he was born." Harvey attributed Parr's death to surfeit and to the pollution of London's air.

The air was certainly as polluted in nineteenth-century Paris as it was in seventeenth-century London. Yet the illustrious French chemist Michel-Eugène Chevreul had reached 103 years of age when he died in 1889, after more than 75 years of residence in the French capital. The photographs taken by Nadar on the occasion of Chevreul's centenary show him to be wiry and spry, as full of *joie de vivre* as a child. When asked how he felt, a short time before his death, he complained only of *une certaine lassitude de vivre*. He was 99 when he published his last scientific paper.

Charles Thierry was born in 1850 and practiced his silversmith trade in Cambridge, Massachusetts, until the age of 93. Every day he took long, vigorous walks in the country, a habit that he kept up after his retirement. At the age of 103 he contracted influenza and had a stormy convalescence. He was then seen by Dr. Paul Dudley White, who urged him to resume his daily walks, regardless of the weather. Thierry recovered but later died of pneumonia at 108 years of age, largely due to his own negligence.

In the 1960s a very old man was brought to New York Hospital from a village in the mountains of Colombia, not for treatment, but for examination by medical scientists, as a curiosity. He was certainly more than 100 years old, and might have been, from circumstantial evidence, approximately 150. He had spent his entire life under primitive conditions, was short and spry, and spoke Spanish with volubility and gusto. I was at the time a patient on the very hospital ward where he was staying as a guest, and can testify to his liveliness, which I greatly envied. He died shortly after returning to Colombia.

In his book, *Old Age,* published in 1904, Elias Metchnikoff presents a cheerful picture of the many very old people he had studied in Russia and in France. According to his accounts, most of them remained active to the very end of their lives, their chief complaint being, as in the case of Chevreul, the kind of lassitude one experiences at the end of a long, full day.

The very existence of healthy, vigorous centenarians, whose lives were spent long before the advent of modern medicine, proves that the potential duration of human existence exceeds the biblical three score and ten, and that longevity can be achieved without medical care. It is probable that the ability to reach a very old age requires a certain genetic constitution, but it is certain that it depends even more on the ways of life. Dr. Alexander Leaf, of Harvard Medical School, has recently made extensive clinical and social observations on very old people in several parts of the world. His studies have led him to suggest that longevity is correlated with a rather frugal diet but of well-balanced composition, vigorous and continued physical activity, and involvement in community affairs to the end of one's life. Complete retirement from active life does not seem to be a good way to reach a very old age.

Healthy centenarians who do not need medical care seem at first sight of no relevance to Norman Cousins's thesis that sick people should share in the responsibility for their treatment. I believe, however, that people can reach a very old age only if they possess some of the physical and psychological attributes that contributed to Cousins's recovery; they must have the will to live that mobilizes the body's natural mechanisms of resistance to disease.

Even under the most urbanized conditions we retain the genetic constitution of our Stone Age ancestors and therefore can never be completely adapted, biologically, to the environments in which we live. Wherever we are and whatever we do, as Cousins says, we cannot avoid being exposed to a multiplicity of physio-chemical and biological agents of disease. We survive only because we are endowed with biological and psychological mechanisms that enable us to respond adaptively to an immense diversity of challenges. This adaptive response may be so effective that most challenges do not result in disease. If disease occurs, the adaptive response commonly brings about spontaneous recovery without the need of medical intervention. Ancient physicians were so familiar with this natural power of the organism to control disease that they invented for it the beautiful expression, *vis medicatrix naturae*, "the healing power of nature."

In his *Anatomy of an Illness*, Cousins identifies the natural recuperative mechanisms of the body with the processes that Walter B. Cannon called homeostatic responses—namely, the natural processes that enable the organism to return to the "normal" state in which it was before being disturbed by a noxious influence. In reality, *vis medicatrix naturae* is much more complex, more powerful and more interesting than Cannon's homeostasis. The response of the organism to disturbances is but rarely homeostatic. Its outcome is more likely to be a lasting change that makes the organism better adapted to future challenges. For example: the development of scar tissue is not a truly homeostatic response; it makes the scarred part of the body better able to resist the insult that caused scarring. Recovery from a given infectious disease is usually accompanied by persistent cellular changes that produce a lasting immunity to that particular infection. Persons who have lost a limb or have become blind tend to develop compensatory skills that become part of their new personality. Instead of being simply homeostatic, the response of the organism corresponds rather to a creative adaptation that is achieved by a permanent change in the body or the mind.

Whether resulting in homeostasis or in creative adaptation, the mechanisms of *vis medicatrix naturae* are so effective that most diseases are self-terminating. Good medical care does of course make the healing process more complete, more rapid and more comfortable, but in the final analysis, as Cousins says, recovery depends upon the mobilization of the patient's own mechanisms of resistance to disease. Herein lies the explanation for the puzzling fact that all ancient and primitive societies have had successful healers, even though medicine had little to offer in the way of really effective therapy until a few decades ago.

Cousins refers to the work of William Osler, who was considered the greatest clinician of the Anglo-

Saxon world at the turn of the century and taught his students that most of the drugs and other methods of treatment available to the physicians of his time were essentially useless. Yet Osler enjoyed an enormous reputation as a healer during his chairmanship of the Department of Medicine at the Johns Hopkins Hospital in Baltimore. On repeated occasions, he expressed the view that the cures of organic diseases he had brought about were due essentially, not to the treatment he used, but to the patient's faith in the effectiveness of the treatment and to the comfort provided by good nursing care. After he had become Regius Professor of Medicine at Oxford University in England, Osler restated once more his conviction that much of his success as a healer was due to aspects of his personality and behavior that were independent of his scientific knowledge of medicine. In an article entitled "The Faith that Heals" he stated amusingly, in 1910, "Our results at the Johns Hopkins Hospital were most gratifying. Faith in *Saint Johns Hopkins*, as we used to call him, an atmosphere of optimism, and cheerful nurses, worked just the same sort of cures as did Aesculapius at Epidaurus" (Osler's italics). When he used the expression "faith healing," Osler referred to the psychological influences that set in motion the restorative mechanisms of *vis medicatrix naturae*—in reality self-healing.

The effectiveness of Osler's "faith healing" was acknowledged even by Dr. William Henry Welch, the main architect of scientific medicine in the United States. Of his father, who practiced medicine in Norfolk, Connecticut, he wrote: "The instant he entered the sick room, the patient felt better. The art of healing seemed to surround his physical body like an aura; it was often not his treatment but his presence that cured." Francis Peabody's famous remark, "The secret of the care of the patient is in caring for the patient," is another way of stating that there is a miraculous moment when the very presence of the doctor is the most effective part of the treatment.

The therapeutic successes of nonmedical healers throughout the ages must be evaluated in the light of the capacity for self-healing that exists in all living forms and particularly in human beings. Although the mechanisms of spontaneous recovery from organic and mental disease are not completely understood, it can be assumed that they all operate through a few common organic pathways and that the organism has only a limited repertoire of responses to healing agencies as diverse as ataractic drugs, the laying on of hands, transcendental meditation, the use of biofeedback techniques, Zen and yoga practices, faith in a saint, a person or a drug—and of course the proper patient-doctor relationship.

Cousins repeatedly states that the mental attitudes of patients have a lot to do with the course of their disease and illustrates this theme with examples taken from clinical material. It is common knowledge, of course, that the mind influences the body and vice versa, but there needs to be more scientific experimentation on this interplay. The examples that I shall mention correspond to different types of immunological and physiological processes which have been studied by the experimental method and which are of a type that can affect the course or the perception of disease.

The body's defense against infection depends in large part on the mechanisms of humoral and cellular immunity, but these mechanisms themselves are influenced by the mental state—as demonstrated by the effect of hypnosis on the Mantoux test. This test consists in the intradermal injection of tuberculin, an extract of tubercle bacilli. It is used to evaluate the likely response of the body to tuberculous infection. A famous English immunologist has recently established, however, that hypnotic suggestion can obliterate the vascular manifestations of the Mantoux test—as neat a proof as one could wish of the influence that the mind exerts over the body. The tuberculin Mantoux reaction pertains to the kind of body response that immunologists designate "cell-mediated immunity." Since this form of the immune response plays an essential role in resistance to important infectious diseases such as tuberculosis, and probably also in resistance to cancer, there is good reason to believe that the patient's state of mind can affect the course of all pathological processes that involve immunological reactions.

The digestion of fats after a meal can be seen as a purely biochemical process involving only the breakdown of the fat particles (chylomicra) by the appropriate enzymes, and the assimilation of the breakdown products into the blood stream and organs, but here again the digestive process is affected by the mind. Observations made on a teacher of anatomy in his forties revealed that the mere prospect of having to lecture to medical students slowed down the rate at which chylomicra disappeared from his blood stream. More generally, it was found that the digestion of fat particles was retarded by almost any disturbance in the life routines. Thus, mental processes can affect the course of physiological processes as seemingly simple as the digestion of food.

Emotional states have long been known to affect the secretion of certain hormones—for example, those of the thyroid and adrenal glands. It has been recently discovered that the brain and the pituitary gland contain a heretofore unknown class of hormones which are chemically related and which go by the collective name endorphins. The physiological activity of some endorphins presents great similarity to that of morphine, heroin, and other opiate substances which relieve pain, not only by acting on the mechanisms of pain itself, but also by inhibiting the emotional response to pain and therefore suffering. Acupuncture can trigger the release of pituitary endorphin which, somehow, gains access to the cells of the spinal cord and can thus exert an opiate-like effect on the perception of pain. It is not too farfetched to assume that, as in the case of other hormones, mental attitudes can affect the secretion of endorphin and thereby the patient's perception of disease.

Cousins correctly points out that a very large percentage of diseases are self-terminating. It can be assumed that much of medical care is useless. In practice, however, most patients can be helped by a physician for several different reasons. Only an accurate diagnosis, arrived at through medical acumen, can determine whether a particular disease is self-terminating or is potentially dangerous and therefore requires a particular therapy. Even in the case of a truly self-terminating disease, professional medical care can hasten the process of recovery and make it more bearable. Furthermore, there are many diseases—hypertension or arthritis, for example—that cannot be cured but for which there exist methods of treatment—medical or surgical—that enable the patient to function more or less normally by correcting the symptoms. Curing the disease is only one aspect of medical care; alleviating the manifestations of disease is often the most important role of the physician.

In view of the diversity of medical intervention, the phrase "good doctor-patient relationships" can be interpreted in several different ways. It can mean that the patient surrenders to the authority of the physician, considered as a father figure. There are many situations in which this type of relationship is necessary, for example in difficult problems of diagnosis or in the application of specific therapies. When I suffered from subacute bacterial endocarditis some seven years ago, the only course for me was to accept the strict regimen of antibiotic therapy which alone can achieve the cure of this otherwise fatal disease. Acceptance of the physician's authority probably facilitates also the operations of what Osler called faith

21

healing, which results in self-healing.

Blind acceptance of the physician's authority, however, seems to be losing ground. Cousins is not the only one to advocate partnership between the physician and patient in the search for a cure. In the summer 1977 issue of *Man and Medicine,* of which Cousins is now advisory editor, Professor Eli Ginzberg of Columbia University states, "No improvement in the health care system will be efficacious unless the citizen assumes responsibility for his own well-being. There are substantial potential gains to be made in linking the individual citizen to the health system through more sophisticated education." In general, the patient's responsibility has been limited to the practice of wiser life styles—giving up smoking, watching one's diet, being more active physically, driving more slowly, learning to live with a chronic ailment such as arthritis or heart disease. But Cousins has a broader view of the patient-physician interplay. According to him, the responsibility of patients goes beyond the practice of healthy ways of life; when possible, it includes sharing with the physician the responsibility for the choice and application of therapy. In my opinion, few are the lay people who can at present usefully take such a creative role in the therapeutic process, except by trying to be objective and truthful in reporting the effects of the treatment. On the other hand, it is all but certain that active participation in the treatment, were it only through laughter or the cultivation of the will to live, as in Cousins's case, helps to mobilize the natural defense mechanisms of the patient which are the indispensable agents of recovery. This is true not only for the cure of an organic disease, but also for reeducation to compensate for a disability of innate or accidental origin. Like cure, rehabilitation implies participation of the mind as well as of the body, integrated through volition for a creative process of adaptive changes.

The questions raised by Cousins should not be read as casting doubts on the validity of scientific medicine. He does not hark back to the days of folk medicine, though he has ample respect for the old-fashioned family doctor. I have always felt that the only trouble with scientific medicine is that it is not scientific enough. Modern medicine will become really scientific only when physicians and their patients have learned to manage the forces of the body and the mind that operate in *vis medicatrix naturae*. This book is a service to that scientific tradition.

# ACKNOWLEDGMENTS

I must begin with my wife, Eleanor, who set me on this path and held me to it.

My debt to Dr. William M. Hitzig is emphasized in the pages that follow. That debt applies not just to the episode described in this book but to more than half a lifetime of friendship and caring.

Hans Selye has been a source of limitless inspiration. Not just as a medical researcher but as a philosopher he has raised the sights of all who know him or have read him. His *From Dream to Discovery* is one of the most exciting intellectual autobiographies it has been my pleasure to read and reflects the creative intelligence at its best. Perhaps it is no accident that it calls to mind *The Way of An Investigator,* by Walter Cannon, who had infinite respect for the drive of the human body to right itself, and who was Selye's teacher. I have a similar missionary zeal about the medical writings of Hans Zinsser, Dana Atchley, and Oliver Wendell Holmes. I am grateful to Lawrence Kubie for his painstaking efforts, many years ago, to impress on me the fact that the greatest advances in medical science will be tied to new knowledge about the workings of the human mind. Jerome Frank, also of Johns Hopkins, has held high Sir William Osler's teachings about the role of faith in healing.

Susan Schiefelbein was of limitless help, especially in providing the research underpinnings and the bibliography for this book. The chapters on "The Mysterious Placebo" and on "What I Learned from Three Thousand Doctors" would not have been possible without her collaboration.

In the preparation of the manuscript and in proofreading, I had the assistance of Emily Suesskind, Mary H. Swift, Shannon Jacobs, and Caroline Blattner, to all of whom I express thanks.

# I

---

# Anatomy of an Illness
# as Perceived by the Patient

This book is about a serious illness that occurred in 1964. I was reluctant to write about it for many years because I was fearful of creating false hopes in others who were similarly afflicted. Moreover, I knew that a single case has small standing in the annals of medical research, having little more than "anecdotal" or "testimonial" value. However, references to the illness surfaced from time to time in the general and medical press. People wrote to ask whether it was true that I "laughed" my way out of a crippling disease that doctors believed to be irreversible. In view of those questions, I thought it useful to provide a fuller account than appeared in those early reports.

In August 1964, I flew home from a trip abroad with a slight fever. The malaise, which took the form of a general feeling of achiness, rapidly deepened. Within a week it became difficult to move my neck, arms, hands, fingers, and legs. My sedimentation rate was over 80. Of all the diagnostic tests, the "sed" rate is one of the most useful to the physician. The way it works is beautifully simple. The speed with which red blood cells settle in a test tube—measured in millimeters per hour—is generally proportionate to the severity of an inflammation or infection. A normal illness, such as grippe, might produce a sedimentation reading of, say, 30 or even 40. When the rate goes well beyond 60 or 70, however, the physician knows that he is dealing with more than a casual health problem. I was hospitalized when the sed rate hit 88. Within a week it was up to 115, generally considered to be a sign of a critical condition.

There were other tests, some of which seemed to me to be more an assertion of the clinical capability of the hospital than of concern for the well-being of the patient. I was astounded when four technicians from four different departments took four separate and substantial blood samples on the same day. That the hospital didn't take the trouble to coordinate the tests, using one blood specimen, seemed to me inexplicable and irresponsible. Taking four large slugs of blood the same day even from a healthy person is hardly to be recommended. When the technicians came the second day to fill their containers with blood for processing in separate laboratories, I turned them away and had a sign posted on my door saying that I would give just one specimen every three days and that I expected the different departments to draw from one vial for their individual needs.

I had a fast-growing conviction that a hospital is no place for a person who is seriously ill. The surprising lack of respect for basic sanitation; the rapidity with which staphylococci and other pathogenic organisms can run through an entire hospital; the extensive and sometimes promiscuous use of X-ray equipment; the seemingly indiscriminate administration of tranquilizers and powerful painkillers, sometimes more for the convenience of hospital staff in managing patients than for therapeutic needs; and the regularity with which hospital routine takes precedence over the rest requirements of the patient (slumber, when it comes for an ill person, is an uncommon blessing and is not to be wantonly interrupted)—all these and other practices seemed to me to be critical shortcomings of the modern hospital.

Perhaps the hospital's most serious failure was in the area of nutrition. It was not just that the meals were poorly balanced; what seemed inexcusable to me was the profusion of processed foods, some of which contained preservatives or harmful dyes. White bread, with its chemical softeners and bleached flour, was offered with every meal. Vegetables were often over-cooked and thus deprived of much of their nutritional value. No wonder the 1969 White House Conference on Food, Nutrition, and Health made the melancholy observation that a great failure of medical schools is that they pay so little attention to the science of nutrition.

My doctor did not quarrel with my reservations about hospital procedures. I was fortunate to have as a physician a man who was able to put himself in the position of the patient. Dr. William Hitzig supported me in the measures I took to fend off the random sanguinary assaults of the hospital laboratory attendants.

We had been close friends for more than twenty years, and he knew of my own deep interest in medical matters. We had often discussed articles in the medical press, including the *New England Journal of Medicine (NEJM)*, and *Lancet*. He was candid with me about my case. He reviewed the reports of the various specialists he had called in as consultants. He said there was no agreement on a precise diagnosis. There was, however, a consensus that I was suffering from a serious collagen illness—a disease of the connective tissue. All arthritic and rheumatic diseases are in this category. Collagen is the fibrous substance that binds the cells together. In a sense, then, I was coming unstuck. I had considerable difficulty in moving my limbs and even in turning over in bed. Nodules appeared on my body, gravel-like substances under the skin, indicating the systemic nature of the disease. At the low point of my illness, my jaws were almost locked.

Dr. Hitzig called in experts from Dr. Howard Rusk's rehabilitation clinic in New York. They confirmed the general opinion, adding the more particularized diagnosis of ankylosing spondylitis, which would mean that the connective tissue in the spine was disintegrating.

I asked Dr. Hitzig about my chances for full recovery. He leveled with me, admitting that one of the specialists had told him I had one chance in five hundred. The specialist had also stated that he had not personally witnessed a recovery from this comprehensive condition.

All this gave me a great deal to think about. Up to that time, I had been more or less disposed to let the doctors worry about my condition. But now I felt a compulsion to get into the act. It seemed clear to me that if I was to be that one in five hundred I had better be something more than a passive observer.

I asked Dr. Hitzig about the possible origin of my condition. He said that it could have come from any one of a number of causes. It could have come, for example, from heavy-metal poisoning, or it could have been the aftereffect of a streptococcal infection.

I thought as hard as I could about the sequence of events immediately preceding the illness. I had gone to the Soviet Union in July 1964 as chairman of an American delegation to consider the problems of cultural exchange. The conference had been held in Leningrad, after which we went to Moscow for supplementary meetings. Our hotel was in a residential area. My room was on the second floor. Each night a procession of diesel trucks plied back and forth to a nearby housing project in the process of round-the-clock construction. It was summer, and our windows were wide open. I slept uneasily each night and felt

31

somewhat nauseated on arising. On our last day in Moscow, at the airport, I caught the exhaust spew of a large jet at point-blank range as it swung around on the tarmac.

As I thought back on that Moscow experience, I wondered whether the exposure to the hydrocarbons from the diesel exhaust at the hotel and at the airport had anything to do with the underlying cause of the illness. If so, that might account for the speculations of the doctors concerning heavy-metal poisoning. The trouble with this theory, however, was that my wife, who had been with me on the trip, had no ill effects from the same exposure. How likely was it that only one of us would have reacted adversely?

It seemed to me, as I thought about it, that there were two possible explanations for the different reactions. One had to do with individual allergy. The second was that I could have been in a condition of adrenal exhaustion and less apt to tolerate a toxic experience than someone whose immunologic system was fully functional.

Was adrenal exhaustion a factor in my own illness?

Again, I thought carefully. The meetings in Leningrad and Moscow had not been casual. Paper work had kept me up late nights. I had ceremonial responsibilities. Our last evening in Moscow had been, at least for me, an exercise in almost total frustration. A reception had been arranged by the chairman of the Soviet delegation at his dacha, located thirty-five to forty miles outside the city. I had been asked if I could arrive an hour early so that I might tell the Soviet delegates something about the individual Americans who were coming to dinner. The Russians were eager to make the Americans feel at home, and they had thought such information would help them with the social amenities.

I was told that a car and driver from the government automobile pool in Moscow would pick me up at the hotel at 3:30 P.M. This would allow ample time for me to drive to the dacha by 5:00, when all our Russian conference colleagues would be gathered for the social briefing. The rest of the American delegation would arrive at the dacha at 6:00 P.M.

At 6:00, however, I found myself in open country on the wrong side of Moscow. There had been a misunderstanding in the transmission of directions to the driver, the result being that we were some eighty miles off course. We finally got our bearings and headed back to Moscow. Our chauffeur had been schooled in cautious driving; he was not disposed to make up lost time. I kept wishing for a driver with a compulsion to prove that auto racing, like baseball, originally came from the U.S.S.R.

We didn't arrive at the dacha until 9:00 P.M. My host's wife looked desolate. The soup had been heated and reheated. The veal was dried out. I felt pretty wrung out myself. It was a long flight back to the States the next day. The plane was overcrowded. By the time we arrived in New York, cleared through the packed customs counters, and got rolling back to Connecticut, I could feel an uneasiness deep in my bones. A week later I was hospitalized.

As I thought back on my experience abroad, I knew that I was probably on the right track in my search for a cause of the illness. I found myself increasingly convinced, as I said a moment ago, that the reason I was hit hard by the diesel and jet pollutants, whereas my wife was not, was that I had had a case of adrenal exhaustion, lowering my resistance.

Assuming this hypothesis was true, I had to get my adrenal glands functioning properly again and to restore what Walter B. Cannon, in his famous book, *The Wisdom of the Body,* called homeostasis.

I knew that the full functioning of my endocrine system—in particular the adrenal glands—was essential for combating severe arthritis or, for that matter, any other illness. A study I had read in the medical press reported that pregnant women frequently have remissions of arthritic or other rheumatic symptoms. The reason is that the endocrine system is fully activated during pregnancy.

How was I to get my adrenal glands and my endocrine system, in general, working well again?

I remembered having read, ten years or so earlier, Hans Selye's classic book, *The Stress of Life.* With great clarity, Selye showed that adrenal exhaustion could be caused by emotional tension, such as frustration or supressed rage. He detailed the negative effects of the negative emotions on body chemistry.

The inevitable question arose in my mind: what about the positive emotions? If negative emotions produce negative chemical changes in the body, wouldn't the positive emotions produce positive chemical changes? Is it possible that love, hope, faith, laughter, confidence, and the will to live have therapeutic value? Do chemical changes occur only on the downside?

Obviously, putting the positive emotions to work was nothing so simple as turning on a garden hose. But even a reasonable degree of control over my emotions might have a salutary physiologic effect. Just replacing anxiety with a fair degree of confidence might be helpful.

A plan began to form in my mind for systematic pursuit of the salutary emotions, and I knew that I would want to discuss it with my doctor. Two preconditions, however, seemed obvious for the experiment. The first concerned my medication. If that medication were toxic to any degree, it was doubtful whether the plan would work. The second precondition concerned the hospital. I knew I would have to find a place somewhat more conducive to a positive outlook on life.

Let's consider these preconditions separately.

First, the medication. The emphasis had been on pain-killing drugs—aspirin, phenylbutazone (butazolidine), codeine, colchicine, sleeping pills. The aspirin and phenylbutazone were antiinflammatory and thus were therapeutically justifiable. But I wasn't sure they weren't also toxic. It developed that I was hypersensitive to virtually all the medication I was receiving. The hospital had been giving me maximum dosages: twenty-six aspirin tablets and twelve phenylbutazone tablets a day. No wonder I had hives all over my body and felt as though my skin were being chewed up by millions of red ants.

It was unreasonable to expect positive chemical changes to take place so long as my body was being saturated with, and toxified by, pain-killing medications. I had one of my research assistants at the *Saturday Review* look up the pertinent references in the medical journals and found that drugs like phenylbutazone and even aspirin levy a heavy tax on the adrenal glands. I also learned that phenylbutazone is one of the most powerful drugs being manufactured. It can produce bloody stools, the result of its antagonism to fibrinogen. It can cause intolerable itching and sleeplessness. It can depress bone marrow.

Aspirin, of course, enjoys a more auspicious reputation, at least with the general public. The prevailing impression of aspirin is that it is not only the most harmless drug available but also one of the most effective. When I looked into research in the medical journals, however, I found that aspirin is quite powerful in its own right and warrants considerable care in its use. The fact that it can be bought in unlimited quantities without prescription or doctor's guidance seemed indefensible. Even in small amounts, it can cause internal bleeding. Articles in the medical press reported that the chemical composition of aspirin, like that of phenylbutazone, impairs the clotting function of platelets, disc-shaped substances in the blood.

It was a mind-boggling train of thought. Could it be, I asked myself, that aspirin, so universally accepted for so many years, was actually harmful in the treatment of collagen illnesses such as arthritis?

The history of medicine is replete with accounts of

drugs and modes of treatment that were in use for many years before it was recognized that they did more harm than good. For centuries, for example, doctors believed that drawing blood from patients was essential for rapid recovery from virtually every illness. Then, midway through the nineteenth century, it was discovered that bleeding served only to weaken the patient. King Charles II's death is believed to have been caused in part by administered bleedings. George Washington's death was also hastened by the severe loss of blood resulting from this treatment.

Living in the second half of the twentieth century, I realized, confers no automatic protection against unwise or even dangerous drugs and methods. Each age has had to undergo its own special nostrums. Fortunately, the human body is a remarkably durable instrument and has been able to withstand all sorts of prescribed assaults over the centuries, from freezing to animal dung.

Suppose I stopped taking aspirin and phenylbutazone? What about the pain? The bones in my spine and practically every joint in my body felt as though I had been run over by a truck.

I knew that pain could be affected by attitudes. Most people become panicky about almost any pain. On all sides they have been so bombarded by advertisements about pain that they take this or that analgesic at the slightest sign of an ache. We are largely illiterate about pain and so are seldom able to deal with it rationally. Pain is part of the body's magic. It is the way the body transmits a sign to the brain that something is wrong. Leprous patients pray for the sensation of pain. What makes leprosy such a terrible disease is that the victim usually feels no pain when his extremities are being injured. He loses his fingers or toes because he receives no warning signal.

I could stand pain so long as I knew that progress was being made in meeting the basic need. That need, I felt, was to restore the body's capacity to halt the continuing breakdown of connective tissue.

There was also the problem of the severe inflammation. If we dispensed with the aspirin, how would we combat the inflammation? I recalled having read in the medical journals about the usefulness of ascorbic acid in combating a wide number of illnesses—all the way from bronchitis to some types of heart disease. Could it also combat inflammation? Did vitamin C act directly, or did it serve as a starter for the body's endocrine system—in particular, the adrenal glands? Was it possible, I asked myself, that ascorbic acid had a vital role to play in "feeding" the adrenal glands?

I had read in the medical press that vitamin C helps to oxygenate the blood. If inadequate or impaired oxygenation was a factor in collagen breakdown, couldn't this circumstance have been another argument for ascorbic acid? Also, according to some medical reports, people suffering from collagen diseases are deficient in vitamin C. Did this lack mean that the body uses up large amounts of vitamin C in the process of combating collagen breakdown?

I wanted to discuss some of these ruminations with Dr. Hitzig. He listened carefully as I told him of my speculations concerning the cause of the illness, as well as my layman's ideas for a course of action that might give me a chance to reduce the odds against my recovery.

Dr. Hitzig said it was clear to him that there was nothing undersized about my will to live. He said that what was most important was that I continue to believe in everything I had said. He shared my excitement about the possibilities of recovery and liked the idea of a partnership.

Even before we had completed arrangements for moving out of the hospital we began the part of the program calling for the full exercise of the affirmative emotions as a factor in enhancing body chemistry. It was easy enough to hope and love and have faith, but what about laughter? Nothing is less funny than being flat on your back with all the bones in your spine and joints hurting. A systematic program was indicated. A good place to begin, I thought, was with amusing movies. Allen Funt, producer of the spoofing television program "Candid Camera," sent films of some of his CC classics, along with a motion-picture projector. The nurse was instructed in its use. We were even able to get our hands on some old Marx Brothers films. We pulled down the blinds and turned on the machine.

It worked. I made the joyous discovery that ten minutes of genuine belly laughter had an anesthetic effect and would give me at least two hours of pain-free sleep. When the pain-killing effect of the laughter wore off, we would switch on the motion-picture projector again, and, not infrequently, it would lead to another pain-free sleep interval. Sometimes, the nurse read to me out of a trove of humor books. Especially useful were E.B. and Katharine White's *Subtreasury of American Humor* and Max Eastman's *The Enjoyment of Laughter.*

How scientific was it to believe that laughter—as well as the positive emotions in general—was affecting my body chemistry for the better? If laughter did in fact have a salutary effect on the body's chemistry, it seemed at least theoretically likely that it would enhance the system's ability to fight the inflammation. So we took sedimentation rate readings just before as well as several hours after the laughter episodes. Each time, there was a drop of at least five points. The drop by itself was not substantial, but it held and was cumulative. I was greatly elated by the discovery that there is a physiologic basis for the ancient theory that laughter is good medicine.

There was, however, one negative side-effect of the laughter from the standpoint of the hospital. I was disturbing other patients. But that objection didn't last very long, for the arrangements were now complete for me to move my act to a hotel room.

One of the incidental advantages of the hotel room, I was delighted to find, was that it cost only about one-third as much as the hospital. The other benefits were incalculable. I would not be awakened for a bed bath or for meals or for medication or for a change of bed sheets or for tests or for examinations by hospital interns. The sense of serenity was delicious and would, I felt certain, contribute to a general improvement.

What about ascorbic acid and its place in the general program for recovery? In discussing my speculations about vitamin C with Dr. Hitzig, I found him completely open-minded on the subject, although he told me of serious questions that had been raised by scientific studies. He also cautioned me that heavy doses of ascorbic acid carried some risk of renal damage. The main problem right then, however, was not my kidneys; it seemed to me that, on balance, the risk was worth taking. I asked Dr. Hitzig about previous recorded experience with massive doses of vitamin C. He ascertained that at the hospital there had been cases in which patients had received up to 3 grams by intramuscular injection.

As I thought about the injection procedure, some questions came to mind. Introducing the ascorbic acid directly into the bloodstream might make more effective use of the vitamin, but I wondered about the body's ability to utilize a sudden, massive infusion. I knew that one of the great advantages of vitamin C is that the body takes only the amount necessary for its purposes and excretes the rest. Again, there came to mind Cannon's phrase—the wisdom of the body.

Was there a coefficient of time in the utilization of ascorbic acid? The more I thought about it, the more likely it seemed to me that the body would excrete a large quantity of the vitamin because it couldn't metabolize it fast enough. I wondered whether a better procedure than injection would be to administer the ascorbic acid through slow intravenous drip over a period of three or four hours. In this way we could go far

41

beyond 3 grams. My hope was to start at 10 grams and then increase the dose daily until we reached 25 grams.

Dr. Hitzig's eyes widened when I mentioned 25 grams. This amount was far beyond any recorded dose. He said he had to caution me about the possible effect not just on the kidneys but on the veins in the arms. Moreover, he said he knew of no data to support the assumption that the body could handle 25 grams over a four-hour period, other than by excreting it rapidly through the urine.

As before, however, it seemed to me we were playing for bigger stakes: losing some veins was not of major importance alongside the need to combat whatever was eating at my connective tissue.

To know whether we were on the right track we took a sedimentation test before the first intravenous administration of 10 grams of ascorbic acid. Four hours later, we took another sedimentation test. There was a drop of nine full points.

Seldom had I known such elation. The ascorbic acid was working. So was laughter. The combination was cutting heavily into whatever poison was attacking the connective tissue. The fever was receding, and the pulse was no longer racing.

We stepped up the dosage. On the second day we went to 12.5 grams of ascorbic acid, on the third day, 15 grams, and so on until the end of the week, when we reached 25 grams. Meanwhile, the laughter routine was in full force. I was completely off drugs and sleeping pills. Sleep—blessed, natural sleep without pain—was becoming increasingly prolonged.

At the end of the eighth day I was able to move my thumbs without pain. By this time, the sedimentation rate was somewhere in the 80s and dropping fast. I couldn't be sure, but it seemed to me that the gravel-like nodules on my neck and the backs of my hands were beginning to shrink. There was no doubt in my mind that I was going to make it back all the way. I could function, and the feeling was indescribably beautiful.

I must not make it appear that all my infirmities disappeared overnight. For many months I couldn't get my arms up far enough to reach for a book on a high shelf. My fingers weren't agile enough to do what I wanted them to do on the organ keyboard. My neck had a limited turning radius. My knees were somewhat wobbly, and off and on, I have had to wear a metal brace.

Even so, I was sufficiently recovered to go back to my job at the *Saturday Review* full time again, and this was miracle enough for me.

Is the recovery a total one? Year by year the mobility has improved. I have become pain-free, except for one shoulder and my knees, although I have been able to discard the metal braces. I no longer feel a sharp twinge in my wrists when I hit a tennis ball or golf ball, as I did for such a long time. I can ride a horse flat out and hold a camera with a steady hand. And I have recaptured my ambition to play the Toccata and Fugue in D Minor, though I find the going slower and tougher than I had hoped. My neck has a full turning radius again, despite the statement of specialists as recently as 1971 that the condition was degenerative and that I would have to adjust to a quarter turn.

It was seven years after the onset of the illness before I had scientific confirmation about the dangers of using aspirin in the treatment of collagen diseases. In its May 8, 1971 issue, *Lancet* published a study by Drs. M. A. Sahud and R. J. Cohen showing that aspirin can be antagonistic to the retention of vitamin C in the body. The authors said that patients with rheumatoid arthritis should take vitamin C supplements, since it has often been noted that they have low levels of the vitamin in their blood. It was no surprise, then, that I had been able to absorb such massive amounts of ascorbic acid without kidney or other complications.

What conclusions do I draw from the entire experience?

The first is that the will to live is not a theoretical abstraction, but a physiologic reality with therapeutic characteristics. The second is that I was incredibly fortunate to have as my doctor a man who knew that his biggest job was to encourage to the fullest the patient's will to live and to mobilize all the natural resources of body and mind to combat disease. Dr. Hitzig was willing to set aside the large and often hazardous armamentarium of powerful drugs available to the modern physician when he became convinced that his patient might have something better to offer. He was also wise enough to know that the art of healing is still a frontier profession. And, though I can't be sure of this point, I have a hunch he believed that my own total involvement was a major factor in my recovery.

People have asked what I thought when I was told by the specialists that my disease was progressive and incurable.

The answer is simple. Since I didn't accept the verdict, I wasn't trapped in the cycle of fear, depression, and panic that frequently accompanies a supposedly incurable illness. I must not make it seem, however, that I was unmindful of the seriousness of the problem or that I was in a festive mood throughout. Being unable to move my body was all the evidence I needed that the specialists were dealing with real concerns. But deep down, I knew I had a good chance and relished the idea of bucking the odds.

Adam Smith, in his book, *Powers of the Mind,* says he discussed my recovery with some of his doctor friends, asking them to explain why the combination of laughter and ascorbic acid worked so well. The answer he got was that neither laughter nor ascorbic acid had anything to do with it and that I probably would have recovered if nothing had been done.

Maybe so, but that was not the opinion of the specialists at the time.

Two or three doctors, reflecting on the Adam Smith account, have commented that I was probably the beneficiary of a mammoth venture in self-administered placebos.

Such a hypothesis bothers me not at all. Respectable names in the history of medicine, like Paracelsus, Holmes, and Osler, have suggested that the history of medication is far more the history of the placebo effect than of intrinsically valuable and relevant drugs. Such modalities as bleeding (in a single year, 1827, France imported 33 million leeches after its domestic supplies had been depleted); purging through emetics; physical contact with unicorn horns, bezoar stones, mandrakes, or powdered mummies—all such treatments were no doubt regarded by physicians at the time as specifics with empirical sanction. But today's medical science recognizes that whatever efficacy these treatments may have had—and the records indicate that the results were often surprisingly in line with expectations—was probably related to the power of the placebo.

Until comparatively recently, medical literature on the phenomenon of the placebo has been rather sparse. But the past two decades have seen a pronounced interest in the subject. Indeed, three medical researchers at the University of California, Los Angeles, have compiled an entire volume on a bibliography of the placebo. (J. Turner, R. Gallimore, C. Fox *Placebo: An Annotated Bibliography*. The Neuropsychiatric Institute, University of California, Los Angeles, 1974.) Among the medical researchers who have been prominently engaged in such studies are Arthur K. Shapiro, Stewart Wolf, Henry K. Beecher, and Louis Lasagna. (Their work is discussed in the next chapter.) In connection with my own experience, I was fascinated by a report citing a study by Dr. Thomas C. Chalmers, of the Mount Sinai Medical Center in New York, which compared two groups that were being used to test the theory that ascorbic acid is a cold preventative. "The group on placebo who thought they were on ascorbic acid," says Dr. Chalmers, "had fewer colds than the group on ascorbic acid who thought they were on placebo."

I was absolutely convinced, at the time I was deep in my illness, that intravenous doses of ascorbic acid could be beneficial—and they were. It is quite possible that this treatment—like everything else I did—was a demonstration of the placebo effect.

At this point, of course, we are opening a very wide door, perhaps even a Pandora's box. The vaunted "miracle cures" that abound in the literature of all the great religions all say something about the ability of the patient, properly motivated or stimulated, to participate actively in extraordinary reversals of disease and disability. It is all too easy, of course, to raise these possibilities and speculations to a monopoly status—in which case the entire edifice of modern medicine would be reduced to little more than the hut of an African witch doctor. But we can at least reflect on William Halse Rivers's statement, as quoted by Shapiro, that "the salient feature of the medicine of today is that these psychical factors are no longer allowed to play their part unwittingly, but are themselves becoming the subject of study, so that the present age is serving the growth of a rational system of psychotherapeutics."

What we are talking about essentially, I suppose, is the chemistry of the will to live. In Bucharest in 1972, I visited the clinic of Ana Aslan, described to me as one of Romania's leading endocrinologists. She spoke of her belief that there is a direct connection between a robust will to live and the chemical balances in the brain. She is convinced that creativity—one aspect of the will to live—produces the vital brain impulses that stimulate the pituitary gland, triggering effects on the pineal gland and the whole of the endocrine system. Is it possible that placebos have a key role in this process? Shouldn't this entire area be worth serious and sustained attention?

If I had to guess, I would say that the principal contribution made by my doctor to the taming, and possibly the conquest, of my illness was that he encouraged me to believe I was a respected partner with him in the total undertaking. He fully engaged my subjective energies. He may not have been able to define or diagnose the process through which self-confidence (wild hunches securely believed) was somehow picked up by the body's immunologic mechanisms and translated into antimorbid effects, but he was acting, I believe, in the best tradition of medicine in recognizing that he had to reach out in my case beyond the usual verifiable modalities. In so doing, he was faithful to the first dictum in his medical education: above all, do not harm.

Something else I have learned. I have learned never to underestimate the capacity of the human mind and body to regenerate—even when the prospects seem most wretched. The life-force may be the least understood force on earth. William James said that human beings tend to live too far within self-imposed limits. It is possible that these limits will recede when we respect more fully the natural drive of the human mind and body toward perfectibility and regeneration. Protecting and cherishing that natural drive may well represent the finest exercise of human freedom.

# 2

---

# The
# Mysterious Placebo

Over long centuries, doctors have been educated by their patients to observe the prescription ritual. Most people seem to feel their complaints are not taken seriously unless they are in possession of a little slip of paper with indecipherable but magic markings. To the patient, a prescription is a certificate of assured recovery. It is the doctor's IOU that promises good health. It is the psychological umbilical cord that provides a nourishing and continuing connection between physician and patient.

The doctor knows that it is the prescription slip itself, even more than what is written on it, that is often the vital ingredient for enabling a patient to get rid of whatever is ailing him. Drugs are not always necessary. Belief in recovery always is. And so the doctor may prescribe a placebo in cases where reassurance for the patient is far more useful than a famous-name pill three times a day.

This strange-sounding word, placebo, is pointing medical science straight in the direction of something akin to a revolution in the theory and practice of medicine. The study of the placebo is opening up vast areas of knowledge about the way the human body heals itself and about the mysterious ability of the brain to order biochemical changes that are essential for combating disease.

The word placebo comes from the Latin verb meaning "I shall please." A placebo in the classical sense, then, is an imitation medicine—generally an innocuous milk-sugar tablet dressed up like an authentic pill—given more for the purpose of placating a patient than for meeting a clearly diagnosed organic need. The placebo's most frequent use in recent years, however, has been in the testing of new drugs. Effects achieved by the preparation being tested are measured against those that follow the administration of a "dummy drug" or placebo.

For a long time, placebos were in general disrepute with a large part of the medical profession. The term, for many doctors, had connotations of quack remedies or "pseudomedicaments." There was also a feeling that placebos were largely a shortcut for some practitioners who were unable to take the time and trouble to get at the real source of a patient's malaise.

Today, however, the once lowly placebo is receiving serious attention from medical scholars. Medical investigators such as Dr. Arthur K. Shapiro, the late Dr. Henry K. Beecher, Dr. Stewart Wolf, and Dr. Louis Lasagna have found substantial evidence that the placebo not only can be made to look like a powerful medication but can actually act like a medication. They regard it not just as a physician's psychological prop in the treatment of certain patients but as an authentic therapeutic agent for altering body chemistry and for helping to mobilize the body's defenses in combating disorder or disease.

While the way the placebo works inside the body is still not completely understood, some placebo researchers theorize that it activates the cerebral cortex, which in turn switches on the endocrine system in general and the adrenal glands in particular. Whatever the precise pathways through the mind and body, enough evidence already exists to indicate that placebos can be as potent as—and sometimes more potent than—the active drugs they replace.

"Placebos," Dr. Shapiro has written in the *American Journal of Psychotherapy,* "can have profound effects on organic illness, including incurable malignancies." One wonders whether this fact may be the key to the puzzle of those cancer sufferers who, according to documented accounts, have recovered after taking Laetril, even though many of the nation's leading cancer research centers have been unable to find any medicinal value in this particular substance.

It is obviously absurd to say that doctors should

never prescribe pharmacologically active drugs. There are times when medication is absolutely essential. But the good doctor is always mindful of its power. No greater popular fallacy exists about medicine than that a drug is like an arrow that can be shot at a particularized target. Its actual effect is more like a shower of porcupine quills. Any drug—or food, for that matter—goes through a process in which the human system breaks it down for use by the whole.

There is almost no drug, therefore, that does not have some side-effects. And the more vaunted the prescription—antibiotics, cortisone, tranquilizers, antihypertensive compounds, antiinflammatory agents, muscle relaxers—the greater the problem of adverse side-effects. Drugs can alter or rearrange the balances in the bloodstream. They can cause the blood to clot faster or slower. They can reduce the level of oxygen in the blood. They can prod the endocrine system, increase the flow of hydrochloric acid to the stomach, slow down or speed up the passage of blood through the heart, impair the blood-making function of the body by depressing the bone marrow, reduce or increase blood pressure, or affect the sodium-potassium exchange, which has a vital part in the body's chemical balance.

The problem posed by many drugs is that they do these things apart from the purpose intended by the physician. There is always the need, therefore, for the doctor to balance off the particularized therapy against the generalized dangers. The more powerful the drug, the more precarious his balancing act.

Complicating the doctor's dilemma about drugs is the fact that many people tend to regard drugs as though they were automobiles. Each year has to have its new models, and the more powerful the better. Too many patients feel the doctor is lacking unless a prescription calls for a new antibiotic or other miracle drug that the patient has heard about from a friend or read about in the press.

Because of the very real dangers associated with powerful new drugs, the prudent modern physician takes full advantage of his freedom of choice, specifying potent drugs when he feels they are absolutely necessary, but disregarding them, prescribing placebos or nothing at all, when they are not.

A hypothetical illustration of how a placebo works is the case of a young businessman who visits his doctor and complains of severe headaches and abdominal pains. After listening carefully to the patient describe not only his pains but his problems, the physician decides that the businessman is suffering from a common disease of the twentieth century: stress. The fact that stress doesn't come from germs or viruses doesn't make its effects any the less serious. Apart from severe illness, it can lead to alcoholism, drug addiction, suicide, family breakdown, joblessness. In extreme form, stress can cause symptoms of conversion hysteria—a malaise described by Jean Charcot, Freud's teacher. The patient's worry and fears are converted into genuine physical symptoms that can be terribly painful or even crippling.

In sympathetic questioning, the doctor learns that

the businessman is worried about the ill health of his pregnant wife and about newly hired young people in his office who seem to him to be angling for his job. The doctor recognizes that his first need is to reassure the patient that nothing is fundamentally wrong with his health. But he is careful not to suggest in any way that the man's pains are unreal or not to be taken seriously. Patients tend to think they have been accused of having imagined their symptoms, of malingering, if their complaint is diagnosed as being psychogenic in origin.

The doctor knows that his patient, in accordance with convention, would probably be uncomfortable without a prescription. But the doctor also knows the limitations of medication. He is reluctant to prescribe tranquilizers because of what he believes would be adverse effects in this particular case. He knows that aspirin would relieve the headaches but would also complicate the gastro-intestinal problem, since even a single aspirin tablet can cause internal bleeding. He rules out digestive aids because he knows that the stomach pains are induced by emotional problems. So the doctor writes a prescription that, first of all, cannot possibly harm the patient and, secondly, might clear up his symptoms. The doctor tells the businessman that the particular prescription will do a great deal of good and that he will recover completely. Then he takes time to discuss with his patient possible ways of meeting the problems at home and at the office.

A week later the businessman telephones the doctor to report that the prescription has worked wonders. The headaches have disappeared and the abdominal pains have lessened. He is less apprehensive about his wife's condition following her visit to the obstetrician, and he seems to be getting along better at the office. How much longer should he take the medicine?

The doctor says that the prescription will probably not have to be refilled but to be sure to telephone if the symptoms recur.

The "wonder" pills, of course, were nothing more than placebos. They had no pharmacological properties. But they worked as well as they did for the businessman because they triggered his body's own ability to right itself, given reasonable conditions of freedom from stress and his complete confidence that the doctor knew what he was doing.

Studies show that up to 90 percent of patients who reach out for medical help are suffering from self-limiting disorders well within the range of the body's own healing powers. The most valuable physician—to a patient and to society—knows how to distinguish effectively between the large number of patients who can get well without heroic intervention and the much smaller number who can't. Such a physician loses no time in mobilizing all the scientific resources and facilities available, but he is careful not to slow up the natural recovery process of those who need his expert reassurance even more than they need his drugs. He may, for such people, prescribe a placebo—both because the patient feels more comfortable with a prescription in his hand and because the doctor knows that the placebo can actually serve a therapeutic purpose.

The placebo, then, is not so much a pill as a process. The process begins with the patient's confidence in the doctor and extends through to the full functioning of his own immunological and healing system. The process works not because of any magic in the tablet but because the human body is its own best apothecary and because the most successful prescriptions are those filled by the body itself.

Berton Roueché, one of America's most talented medical reporters, wrote an article for the *New Yorker* magazine in 1960 in which he said that the placebo derives its power from the "infinite capacity of the human mind for self-deception." This interpretation is not held by placebo scholars. They believe that the placebo is powerful not because it "fools" the body but because it translates the will to live into a physical reality. And they have been able to document the fact that the placebo triggers specific biochemical changes in the body. The fact that a placebo will have no physiological effect if the patient knows it is a placebo only confirms something about the capacity of the human body to transform hope into tangible and essential biochemical change.

The placebo is proof that there is no real separation between mind and body. Illness is always an interaction between both. It can begin in the mind and affect the body, or it can begin in the body and affect the mind, both of which are served by the same bloodstream. Attempts to treat most mental diseases as though they were completely free of physical causes and attempts to treat most bodily diseases as though the mind were in no way involved must be considered archaic in the light of new evidence about the way the human body functions.

Placebos will not work under all circumstances. The chances of successful use are believed to be directly proportionate to the quality of a patient's relationship with a doctor. The doctor's attitude toward the patient; his ability to convince the patient that he is not being taken lightly; his success in gaining the full confidence of the patient—all these are vital factors not just in maximizing the usefulness of a placebo but in the treatment of illness in general. In the absence of a strong relationship between doctor and patient, the use of placebos may have little point or prospect. In this sense, the doctor himself is the most powerful placebo of all.

A striking example of the doctor's role in making a placebo work can be seen in an experiment in which patients with bleeding ulcers were divided into two groups. Members of the first group were informed by the doctor that a new drug had just been developed that would undoubtedly produce relief. The second group was told by nurses that a new experimental drug would be administered, but that very little was known about its effects. Seventy percent of the people in the first group received sufficient relief from their ulcers. Only 25 percent of the patients in the second group experienced similar benefit. Both groups had been given the identical "drug"—a placebo.

How much scientific laboratory data has been accumulated on placebo efficacy? The medical literature in the past quarter-century contains an impressive number of cases:

The late Dr. Henry K. Beecher, noted anesthesiologist at Harvard, considered the results of fifteen studies involving 1,082 patients. He discovered that across the broad spectrum of these tests, 35 percent of the patients consistently experienced "satisfactory relief" when placebos were used instead of regular medication for a wide range of medical problems, including severe postoperative wound pain, seasickness, headaches, coughs, and anxiety. Other biological processes and disorders affected by placebos, as reported by medical researchers, include rheumatoid and degenerative arthritis, blood-cell count, respiratory rates, vasomotor function, peptic ulcers, hay fever, hypertension, and spontaneous remission of warts.

Dr. Stewart Wolf wrote that placebo effects are "neither imaginary nor necessarily suggestive in the usual sense of the word." His comments were connected to the results of a test in which specialized blood cells called eosinophils accumulate beyond their normal numbers and circulate throughout the system. The test showed that placebos can change body chemistry. Wolf also reported a test by a colleague in which a placebo reduced the amount of fat and protein in the blood.

When a patient suffering from Parkinson's disease was given a placebo but was told he was receiving a drug, his tremors decreased markedly. After the effects of the placebo wore off, the same substance was put into his milk without his knowledge. The tremors reappeared.

During a large study of mild mental depression, patients who had been treated with sophisticated stimulants were taken off the drugs and put on placebos. The patients showed exactly the same improvement as they had gained from the drugs. In a related study doctors gave placebos to 133 depressed patients who had not yet received a drug. One-quarter of them responded so well to placebos that they were excluded from further testing of actual drugs.

When a group of patients were given a placebo in place of an antihistamine, 77.4 percent reported drowsiness, which is characteristic of antihistamine drugs.

In a study of postoperative wound pain by Beecher and Lasagna, a group of patients who had just undergone surgery were alternately given morphine and placebos. Those who took morphine immediately after surgery registered a 52-percent relief factor; those who took the placebo first, 40 percent. The placebo was 77 percent as effective as morphine. Beecher and Lasagna also discovered that the more severe the pain, the more effective the placebo.

Eighty-eight arthritic patients were given placebos instead of aspirin or cortisone. The number of patients who benefited from the placebos was approximately the same as the number benefiting from the conventional antiarthritic drugs. Some of the patients who had experienced no relief from the placebo tablets were given placebo injections. Sixty-four percent of those given injections reported relief and improvement. For the entire group, the benefits included not just pain relief but general improvement in eating, sleeping, elimination, and even reduction in swelling.

A. Leslie reported that morphine addicts have been given placebos (saline injections) and have not suffered withdrawal symptoms until the injections were stopped.

A group of medical students were invited to participate in an experiment they were told was for the purpose of testing the efficacy of a depressant and a stimulant. They were informed in detail of the effects, beneficial and adverse, that could be expected from these drugs. They were not told that both "stimulants" and "depressants" were actually placebos. More than half the students exhibited specific physiological reactions to the placebos. The pulse rate fell in 66 percent of the subjects. A decrease in arterial pressure was observed in 71 percent of the students. Adverse side effects included dizziness, abdominal stress, and watery eyes.

Medical officials of the National Institute of Geriatrics in Bucharest, Romania, undertook a double-blind experiment to test a new drug designed to activate the endocrine system and thus enhance health and the prospects for increased longevity. A total of 150 Romanians sixty years of age, all of whom lived under approximately the same village conditions, were divided into three groups of 50 each. The first group received nothing. The second group received a placebo. The third was given regular treatment with the new drug. Year by year, all three groups were carefully observed with respect to mortality and morbidity. The statistics for the first group conformed with those for other Romanian villagers of similar age. The second group, on the placebo, showed a marked improvement in health and a measurably lower death rate than the first group. The third group, on the drug, showed about the same improvement over the placebo group as the placebo group showed over the first.

If the placebo can do a great deal of good, it can also do a great deal of harm. The cerebral cortex stimulates negative biochemical changes just as it does positive changes. Beecher stressed as long ago as 1955, in the *Journal of the American Medical Association,* that placebos can have serious toxic effects and produce physiological damage. A case in point is a study of the drug mephenesin's effect on anxiety. In some patients, it produces such adverse reactions as nausea, dizziness, and palpitation. When a placebo was substituted for mephenesin, it produced identical reactions in an identical percentage of doses. One of the patients, after taking the placebo, developed a skin rash that disappeared immediately after placebo administration was stopped. Another collapsed in anaphylatic shock when she took the drug. A third experienced abdominal pain and a build-up of fluid in her hips within ten minutes after taking the placebo—before she had even taken the drug.

It would be reasonable to conclude from the foregoing that the placebo effect applies to all drugs in varying degrees. Indeed, many medical scholars have believed that the history of medicine is actually the history of the placebo effect. Sir William Osler underlined the point by observing that the human species is distinguished from the lower orders by its desire to take medicine. Considering the nature of nostrums taken over the centuries, it is possible that another distinguishing feature of the species is its ability to survive medication. At various times and in various places, prescriptions have called for animal dung, powdered mummies, sawdust, lizard's blood, dried vipers, sperm from frogs, crab's eyes, weed roots, sea sponges, "unicorn horns," and lumpy substances extracted from the intestines of cud-chewing animals.

Pondering this grim array of potions and procedures, which were as medically respectable in their day as any of the vaunted medicines in use today, Dr. Shapiro has commented that "one may wonder how physicians maintained their positions of honor and respect throughout history in the face of thousands of years of prescribing useless and often dangerous medications."

The answer is that people were able to overcome these noxious prescriptions, along with the assorted malaises for which they had been prescribed, because their doctors had given them something far more valuable than the drugs: a robust belief that what they were getting was good for them. They had reached out to their doctors for help; they believed they were going to be helped—and they were.

Some people are more susceptible to placebo therapy than others. Why? It used to be assumed that there was some correlation between high suggestibility and low intelligence, and that people with low IQs were therefore apt to be better placebo subjects. This theory was exploded by Dr. H. Gold at the Cornell Conference on Therapy in 1946. The higher the intelligence, said Dr. Gold on the basis of his extended studies, the greater the potential benefit from the use of placebos.

Inevitably, the use of the placebo involved built-in contradictions. A good patient-doctor relationship is essential to the process, but what happens to that relationship when one of the partners conceals important information from the other? If the doctor tells the truth, he destroys the base on which the placebo rests. If he doesn't tell the truth, he jeopardizes a relationship built on trust.

This dilemma poses a question involving medical ethics: when is a physician justified in not being completely candid with the patient? In terminal cases, the doctor may think it unwise and even irresponsible to add desolation to pain: and so he skirts around the truth. What about drug addiction? Placebos are now being used by some doctors as a substitute for hard drugs in a systematic attempt to wean their patients away from addiction. In these cases, the patient exhibits the same solution as he does to heroin or cocaine. The body's raging desire for the drug is appeased—but it doesn't pay the physiological price of the addictive poisons. Should doctors withhold such treatment because they feel it is a breach of medical ethics not to inform the patient about the true nature of the treatment?

In an even more fundamental sense, it may be asked whether it is ethical—or, what is more important, wise—for the doctor to nourish the patient's mystical belief in medication. An increasing number of doctors believe they should not encourage their patients to expect prescriptions, for they know how easy it is to deepen the patient's psychological and physiological dependence on drugs—or even on placebos, for that matter. Such an approach carries with it the risk that the patient will go across the street to another doctor; but if enough doctors break with ritual in this respect, there is hope that the patient himself will regard the prescription slip in a new light. Dr. Richard C. Cabot once wrote that "the patient has learned to expect a medicine for every symptom. He was not born with that expectation. . . . It is we physicians who are responsible for perpetuating false ideas about disease and its cure."

Another problem in medical ethics arises because many doctors believe not enough is known about the effects of the placebo on the delicate structure and functions of the body's nervous system. Should the benefits of the placebo be deferred until such time as more answers are obtained?

Certainly the medical profession is not without precedent in the use of modalities or drugs about which full knowledge is still absent. Electric shock is being used in the treatment of mental disease even though doctors don't know exactly what happens inside the brain when it is jolted by high voltage. The most widely used drug in the world is aspirin, yet why it reduces inflammation is a mystery.

True, not everything is known about the placebo. But enough is known to put its continued study high on the medical and human agenda. Knowing more about the gift of life is not merely a way of satisfying random curiosity. In the end, it is what education is all about.

The most prevalent—and, for all we know, most serious—health problem of our time is stress, which is defined by Hans Selye, dean of the stress concept, as the "rate of wear and tear in the human body." This definition would thus embrace any demands, whether emotional or physical, beyond the ready capability of any given individual.

The war against microbes has been largely won, but the struggle for equanimity is being lost. It is not just the congestion outside us—a congestion of people and ideas and issues—but our inner congestion that is hurting us. Our experiences come at us in such profusion and from so many different directions that they are never really sorted out, much less absorbed. The result is clutter and confusion. We gorge the senses and starve the sensitivities.

"Your health is bound to be affected," Boris Pasternak wrote in *Dr. Zhivago*, "if, day after day, you say the opposite of what you feel, if you grovel before what you dislike and rejoice at what brings you nothing but misfortune. Our nervous system isn't just a fiction; it's a part of our physical body, and our soul exists in space, and is inside us, like the teeth in our mouth. It can't be forever violated with impunity. I found it painful to listen to you, Innokentii, when you told us how you were re-educated and became mature in jail. It was like listening to a horse describing how it broke itself in."

It is doubtful whether the placebo—or any drug, for that matter—would get very far without a patient's robust will to live. For the will to live is a window on the future. It opens the individual to such help as the outside world has to offer, and it connects that help to the body's own capability for fighting disease. It enables the human body to make the most of itself. The placebo has a role to play in transforming the will to live from a poetical conception to a physical reality and a governing force.

In the end, the greatest value of the placebo is what it can tell us about life. Like a celestial chaperon, the placebo leads us through the uncharted passageways of mind and gives us a greater sense of infinity than if we were to spend all our days with our eyes hypnotically glued to the giant telescope at Mt. Palomar. What we see ultimately is that the placebo isn't really necessary and that the mind can carry out its difficult and wondrous missions unprompted by little pills. The placebo is only a tangible object made essential in an age that feels uncomfortable with intangibles, an age that prefers to think that every inner effect must have an outer cause. Since it has size and shape and can be hand-held, the placebo satisfies the contemporary craving for visible mechanisms and visible answers. But the placebo dissolves on scrutiny, telling us that it cannot relieve us of the need to think deeply about ourselves.

The placebo, then, is an emissary between the will to live and the body. But the emissary is expendable. If we can liberate ourselves from tangibles, we can connect hope and the will to live directly to the ability of the body to meet great threats and challenges. The mind can carry out its ultimate functions and powers over the body without the illusion of material intervention. "The mind," said John Milton, "is its own place, and in itself can make a heaven of hell, and a hell of heaven."

Science is concocting exotic terms like biofeedback to describe the control by the mind over the autonomic nervous system. But labels are unimportant; what is important is the knowledge that human beings are not locked into fixed limitations. The quest for perfectibility is not a presumption or a blasphemy but the highest manifestation of a great design.

Some years ago, I had an opportunity to observe African witch-doctor medicine at first hand in the Gabon jungle country. At the dinner table of the Schweitzer Hospital at Lambarene, I had ventured the remark that the local people were lucky to have access to the Schweitzer clinic instead of having to depend on witch-doctor supernaturalism. Dr. Schweitzer asked me how much I knew about witch doctors. I was trapped by my ignorance—and we both knew it. The next day *le grand docteur* took me to a nearby jungle clearing, where he introduced me to *un de mes collègues*, an elderly witch doctor. After a respectful exchange of greetings, Dr. Schweitzer suggested that his American friend be allowed to observe African medicine.

For the next two hours, we stood off to one side and watched the witch doctor at work. With some patients, the witch doctor merely put herbs in a brown paper bag and instructed the ill person in their use. With other patients, he gave no herbs but filled the air with incantations. A third category of patients he merely spoke to in a subdued voice and pointed to Dr. Schweitzer.

On our way back to the clinic, Dr. Schweitzer explained what had happened. The people who had assorted complaints that the witch doctor was able to diagnose readily were given special herbs to make into brews. Dr. Schweitzer guessed that most of those patients would improve very rapidly since they had only functional, rather than organic, disturbances. Therefore, the "medications" were not really a major factor. The second group had psychogenic ailments that were being treated with African psychotherapy. The third group had more substantial physical problems, such as massive hernias or extrauterine pregnancies or dislocated shoulders or tumorous conditions. Many of these problems required surgery, and the witch doctor was redirecting the patients to Dr. Schweitzer himself.

"Some of my steadiest customers are referred to me by witch doctors," Dr. Schweitzer said with only the slightest trace of a smile. "Don't expect me to be too critical of them."

When I asked Dr. Schweitzer how he accounted

for the fact that anyone could possibly expect to become well after having been treated by a witch doctor, he said that I was asking him to divulge a secret that doctors have carried around inside them ever since Hippocrates.

"But I'll tell you anyway," he said, his face still illuminated by that half-smile. "The witch doctor succeeds for the same reason all the rest of us succeed. Each patient carries his own doctor inside him. They come to us not knowing that truth. We are at our best when we give the doctor who resides within each patient a chance to go to work."

The placebo is the doctor who resides within.

# 3

---

# Creativity
# and Longevity

What started me thinking about creativity and longevity, and the connection between the two, were examples of two men who were very much alike in vital respects: Pablo Casals and Albert Schweitzer.

Both were octogenarians when I met them for the first time. Both were fully creative—almost explosively so. Both were committed to personal undertakings that were of value to other human beings. What I learned from these two men had a profound effect on my life—especially during the period of my illness. I learned that a highly developed purpose and the will to live are among the prime raw materials of human existence. I became convinced that these materials may well represent the most potent force within human reach.

First, some observations about Pablo Casals.

I met him for the first time at his home in Puerto Rico just a few weeks before his ninetieth birthday. I was fascinated by his daily routine. About 8 A.M. his lovely young wife Marta would help him to start the day. His various infirmities made it difficult for him to dress himself. Judging from his difficulty in walking and from the way he held his arms, I guessed he was suffering from rheumatoid arthritis. His emphysema was evident in his labored breathing. He came into the living room on Marta's arm. He was badly stooped. His head was pitched forward and he walked with a shuffle. His hands were swollen and his fingers were clenched.

Even before going to the breakfast table, Don Pablo went to the piano — which, I learned, was a daily ritual. He arranged himself with some difficulty on the piano bench, then with discernible effort raised his swollen and clenched fingers above the keyboard.

I was not prepared for the miracle that was about to happen. The fingers slowly unlocked and reached toward the keys like the buds of a plant toward the sunlight. His back straightened. He seemed to breathe more freely. Now his fingers settled on the keys. Then came the opening bars of Bach's *Wohltemperierte Klavier*, played with great sensitivity and control. I had forgotten that Don Pablo had achieved proficiency on several musical instruments before he took up the cello. He hummed as he played, then said that Bach spoke to him here—and he placed his hand over his heart.

Then he plunged into a Brahms concerto and his fingers, now agile and powerful, raced across the keyboard with dazzling speed. His entire body seemed fused with the music; it was no longer stiff and shrunken but supple and graceful and completely freed of its arthritic coils.

Having finished the piece, he stood up by himself, far straighter and taller than when he had come into the room. He walked to the breakfast table with no trace of a shuffle, ate heartily, talked animatedly, finished the meal, then went for a walk on the beach.

After an hour or so, he came back to the house and worked on his correspondence until lunch. Then he napped. When he rose, the stoop and the shuffle and the clenched hands were back again. On this particular day, a camera and recording crew from public television were scheduled to arrive in mid-afternoon. Anticipating the visit, Don Pablo said he wished some way could be found to call it off; he didn't feel up to the exertion of the filming, with its innumerable and inexplicable retakes and the extreme heat of the bright lights.

Marta, having been through these reluctances before, reassured Don Pablo, saying she was certain he would be stimulated by the meeting. She reminded him that he liked the young people who did the last filming and that they would probably be back again. In particular, she called his attention to the lovely young lady who directed the recording.

Don Pablo brightened. "Yes, of course," he said, "it will be good to see them again."

As before, he stretched his arms in front of him and extended his fingers. Then the spine straightened and he stood up and went to his cello. He began to play. His fingers, hands, and arms were in sublime coordination as they responded to the demands of his brain for the controlled beauty of movement and tone. Any cellist thirty years his junior would have been proud to have such extraordinary physical command.

Twice in one day I had seen the miracle. A man almost ninety, beset with the infirmities of old age, was able to cast off his afflictions, at least temporarily, because he knew he had something of overriding importance to do. There was no mystery about the way it worked, for it happened every day. Creativity for Pablo Casals was the source of his own cortisone. It is doubtful whether any antiinflammatory medication he would have taken would have been as powerful or as safe as the substances produced by the interaction of his mind and body.

The process is not strange. If he had been caught up in an emotional storm, the effects would have been manifested in an increased flow of hydrochloric acid to the stomach, in an upsurge of adrenal activity, in the production of corticoids, in the increase of blood pressure, and a faster heart beat.

But he was caught up in something else. He was caught up in his own creativity, in his own desire to accomplish a specific purpose, and the effect was both genuine and observable. And the effects on his body chemistry were no less pronounced—albeit in a positive way—than they would have been if he had been through an emotional wringer.

* * *

Don Pablo, though delicately built, almost frail, was a giant among men in spirit and creative stature. He was buoyantly sympathetic in manner, managing to involve himself very quickly in the concerns or problems of his friends or visitors. His responses were unhurried, genuine, full. He showed me some of his original Bach manuscripts, and he remarked that Bach meant more to him than any other composer.

This was only one of several things he had in common with Schweitzer, I remarked.

"My good friend Albert Schweitzer shares with me the belief that Bach is the greatest of all composers," Don Pablo said, "but we like Bach for entirely different reasons. Schweitzer sees Bach in complex architectural terms; he acclaims him as a master who reigns supreme over the great and diverse realm of music. I see Bach as a great romantic. His music stirs me, helps me to feel fully alive. When I wake up each morning I can hardly wait to play Bach. What a wonderful way to start the day."

If Bach was his favorite composer, what was his favorite composition?

"The piece that means the most to me was written not by Bach but by Brahms," he said. "Here, let me show it to you. I have the original manuscript."

He took down from the wall, where it had been framed behind glass, one of the most valuable music manuscripts in the world now in private hands—Brahms's B-flat Quartet.

"Interesting, how I happened to acquire it," he said. "Many years ago I knew a man who was head of the Friends of Music in Vienna. His name was Wilhelm Kuchs. One night in Vienna—this was before the war—he invited several of his friends for dinner, myself included. He had what I believe may have been the finest private collection of original music manuscripts in the world. He also owned an impressive collection of fine musical instruments—violins by Stradivarius and Guarneri among them. He was wealthy, very wealthy, but he was a simple man and a very accessible one.

"Then the war came. He was in his eighties. He had no intention of spending the rest of his old age under Nazism. He moved to Switzerland. He was then more than ninety. I was eager to pay my respects. Just seeing him again, this wonderful old friend who had done so much for music, was to me a very moving experience. I think we both wept on each other's shoulder. Then I told him how concerned I had been over this collection of manuscripts. I had been terribly apprehensive that he might not have been able to keep his collection from falling into Nazi hands.

"My friend told me there was nothing to worry about; he had managed to save the entire collection. Then he went and got some items from the collection

—some chamber music by Schubert and Mozart to begin with. Then he placed on the table before me the original manuscript of the Brahms B-flat Quartet. I could hardly believe my eyes. I stood transfixed. I suppose every musician feels that there is one piece that speaks to him alone, one which he feels seems to involve every molecule of his being. This was the way I had felt about the B-flat Quartet ever since I played it for the first time. And always I felt it was mine.

"Mr. Kuchs could see that when I held the B-flat Quartet manuscript in my hands it was a very special and powerful emotional experience.

" 'It is *your* quartet in every way,' Mr. Kuchs said. 'It would make me happy if you would let me give it to you.' And he did.

"I couldn't thank him adequately then, but I did write him a long letter telling him of the great pride and joy his gift had brought to my life. When Mr. Kuchs replied, he told me many things about the history of the B-flat Quartet I had not known before. One fact in particular stood out. It is that Brahms began to write the quartet just nine months before I was born. It took him nine months to complete it. We both came into the world on exactly the same day, the same month, the same year."

As Don Pablo spoke, he seemed to relive the experience. His features, unmarred by any hard lines, were so expressive that his words seemed merely to confirm the image. Indeed, his face had the dramatic power of a full Ibsen cast.

I asked Don Pablo whether any other individual

compositions had special meaning for him.

"Many pieces," he said, "but none that I felt owned me and expressed me as much as the B-flat Quartet. Yet, when I get up in the morning, I can think only of Bach. I have the feeling that the world is being reborn. Nature always seems more in evidence to me in the morning.

"There is one other piece I must tell you about. This one, too, has special meaning. I think it is the piece I would like most to hear again during my last moments on earth. How lovely and moving it is, the second movement of Mozart's Clarinet Quintet."

Don Pablo played it. His fingers were thin and the skin was pale but they belonged to the most extraordinary hands I had ever seen. They seemed to have a wisdom and a grace of their own. When he played Mozart, he was clearly the interpreter and not just the performer; yet it was difficult to imagine how the piece could be played in any other way.

After he got up from the piano he apologized for having taken up so much time in our talk with music, instead of discussing the affairs of the world. I told him I had the impression that what he had been saying and doing were most relevant in terms of the world's affairs. In the discussion that followed there seemed to be agreement on the proposition that the most serious part of the problem of world peace was that the individual felt helpless.

"The answer to helplessness is not so very complicated." Don Pablo said. "A man can do something for peace without having to jump into politics. Each man has inside him a basic decency and goodness. If he listens to it and acts on it, he is giving a great deal of what it is the world needs most. It is not complicated but it takes courage. It takes courage for a man to listen to his own goodness and act on it. Do we dare to be ourselves? This is the question that counts."

The decency and goodness within Don Pablo were clearly evident. But there were other resources—purpose, the will to live, faith, and good humor—that enabled him to cope with his infirmities and to perform as cellist and conductor well into his nineties.

*  *  *

Albert Schweitzer always believed that the best medicine for any illness he might have was the knowledge that he had a job to do, plus a good sense of humor. He once said that disease tended to leave him rather rapidly because it found so little hospitality inside his body.

The essence of Dr. Schweitzer was purpose and creativity. All his multiple skills and interests were energized by a torrential drive to use his mind and body. To observe him at work at his hospital in Lambarene was to see human purpose bordering on the supernatural. During an average day at the hospital, even after he turned ninety, he would attend to his duties at the clinic and make his rounds, do strenuous carpentry, move heavy crates of medicine, work on his correspondence (innumerable letters each day), give time to his unfinished manuscripts, and play the piano.

"I have no intention of dying," he once told his staff, "so long as I can do things. And if I do things, there is no need to die. So I will live a long, long time."

And he did–until he was ninety-five.

Like his friend Pablo Casals, Albert Schweitzer would not allow a single day to pass without playing Bach. His favorite piece was the Toccata and Fugue in D Minor. The piece was written for the organ. But there were no organs in Lambarene. There were two pianos, both uprights, both ancient. The one in the staff dining room was the more battered of the two. The equatorial climate, with its saturating humidity, had vanquished it almost beyond recognition. Some of the keys had no ivories; others were yellowed and cracked. The felt on the hammers had worn thin and produced harsh, twanging sounds. The instrument hadn't been tuned in years; even if it had been, the improvement would have been short-lived. On my first visit to the hospital, I wandered into the dining room, sat down to play, then drew back abruptly at the caricatured tones. Yet the amazing thing was that Schweitzer could play hymns on it at dinner time each evening and the piano somehow lost its poverty in his hands.

The other piano was in his bungalow. It was in far better shape than the one in the dining room but it was hardly what one would call playable for a performer of Schweitzer's worldwide reputation. It had an organ footboard attachment that was engineered into the hammer action, but this footboard had the infuriating habit of becoming detached in the middle of critical passages. Even a phantom footboard, however, provided him with an opportunity to work his feet.

In an earlier book, I wrote about my experience at the Lambarene hospital when, one night, long after most of the oil lamps had been turned out, I walked down toward the river. It was a sticky night and I couldn't sleep. As I passed the compound near Dr. Schweitzer's quarters, I could hear the rapid piano movement of a Bach toccata.

I approached the doctor's bungalow and stood for perhaps five minutes outside the latticed window, through which I could see his silhouette at the piano in the dimly lit room. His powerful hands were in total control of the composition and he met Bach's demands for complete definition of each note—each with its own weight and value, yet all of them intimately interlaced to create an ordered whole.

I had a stronger sense of listening to a great console than if I had been in the world's largest cathedral. The yearning for an architectured beauty in music; the disciplined artistry and the palpable desire to keep alive a towering part of his past; the need for outpouring and catharsis—all these things inside Albert Schweitzer spoke in his playing.

And when he was through he sat with his hands resting lightly on the keys, his great head bent forward as though to catch the lingering echoes. Johann

Sebastian Bach had made it possible for him to free himself of the pressures and tensions of the hospital, with its forms to fill out in triplicate. He was now restored to the world of creative and ordered splendor that he had always found in music.

The effect of the music was much the same on Schweitzer as it had been on Casals. He felt restored, regenerated, enhanced. When he stood up, there was no trace of a stoop. Music was his medicine.

But not the only medicine. There was also humor.

Albert Schweitzer employed humor as a form of equatorial therapy, a way of reducing the temperatures and the humidity and the tensions. His use of humor, in fact, was so artistic that one had the feeling he almost regarded it as a musical instrument.

Life for the young doctors and nurses was not easy at the Schweitzer Hospital. Dr. Schweitzer knew it and gave himself the task of supplying nutrients for their spirits. At mealtimes, when the staff came together, Schweitzer always had an amusing story or two to go with the meal. Laughter at the dinner hour was probably the most important course. It was fascinating to see the way the staff members seemed to be rejuvenated by the wryness of his humor. At one meal, for example, Dr. Schweitzer reported to the staff that, "as everyone knows, there are only two automobiles within seventy-five miles of the hospital. This afternoon, the inevitable happened; the cars collided. We have treated the drivers for their superficial wounds. Anyone who has reverence for machines may treat the cars."

The next evening, he passed along the news that six baby chicks had been born to Edna the hen, who made her home near the dock. "It was a great surprise to me," he said solemnly, "I didn't even know she was that way."

One night at the dinner table, after a particularly trying day, he related to the staff an account of his visit to the Royal Palace in Copenhagen some years earlier. The invitation was for dinner, the first course of which was Danish herring. Schweitzer didn't happen to like herring. When no one was looking he deftly slipped the herring off the plate and into his jacket pocket. The next day, one of the local newspapers, reporting on the life at the Royal Palace, told of the visit of the jungle doctor and of the strange eating habits he had picked up in Africa. Not only did Dr. Schweitzer eat the meat of the fish, the newspaper reported; he ate the bones, head, eyes and all.

I noticed that when the young doctors and nurses got up from the table that evening, they were in a fine mood, refreshed as much by the spirit of the occasion as by the food. Dr. Schweitzer's fatigue, so palpable when he first came into the dining room, now gave way to anticipations of things that had to be done. Humor at Lambarene was vital nourishment.

The Bible tells us that a merry heart works like a doctor. Exactly what happens inside the human mind and body as the result of humor is difficult to say. But the evidence that it works has stimulated the speculations not just of physicians but of philosophers and scholars over the centuries. Sir Francis Bacon called attention to the physiological characteristics of mirth. Robert Burton, in his *Anatomy of Melancholy*, almost four hundred years ago, cited authorities for his observation that "humor purges the blood, making the body young, lively, and fit for any manner of employment." In general, Burton said, mirth is the "principal engine for battering the walls of melancholy . . . and a sufficient cure in itself." Hobbes described laughter as a "passion of sudden glory."

Immanuel Kant, in his *Critique of Pure Reason*, wrote that laughter produces a "feeling of health through the furtherance of the vital bodily processes, the affection that moves the intestines and the diaphragms; in a word, the feeling of health that makes up the gratification felt by us; so that we can thus reach the body through the soul and use the latter as the physician of the former." If Kant was intimating in these remarks that he never knew a man who possessed the gift of hearty laughter to be burdened by constipation, I can readily agree with him. It has always seemed to me that hearty laughter is a good way to jog internally without having to go outdoors.

Sigmund Freud's fascination with the human mind was not confined to its malfunctioning or its torments. His researches were directed to the supremely mysterious station occupied by the brain in the universe. Wit and humor to him were highly differentiated manifestations of the uniqueness of the mind. He believed that mirth was a highly useful way of counteracting nervous tension, and that humor could be used as effective therapy.

Sir William Osler regarded laughter as the "music of life." His biographer, Harvey Cushing, quoted Osler as having advised doctors who are spiritually and physically depleted at the end of a long day to find their own medicine in mirth. "There is the happy possibility," Osler wrote, "that like Lionel in, I think, one of Shelley's poems, he may keep himself young with laughter."

Current scientific research in the physiological benefits of laughter may not be abundant but is significant nonetheless. William Fry, of Stanford University, has written a highly illuminating paper, "The Respiratory Components of Mirthful Laughter." I assume he is referring to what is commonly known as belly laughter. Like Immanuel Kant, Fry finds that the entire process of respiration is benevolently engaged by laughter. Another paper worth consulting on the subject is "Effect of Laughter on Muscle Tone," written by H. Paskind in the *Archives of Neurology and Psychiatry* in 1932.

Some people, in the grip of uncontrollable laughter, say their ribs are hurting. The expression is probably accurate, but it is a delightful "hurt" that leaves the individual relaxed almost to the point of an open sprawl. It is the kind of "pain," too, that most people would do well to experience every day of their lives. It is as specific and tangible as any other form of physical exercise. Though its biochemical manifestations have yet to be as explicitly charted and understood as the effects of fear or frustration or rage, they are real enough.

Increasingly, in the medical press, articles are being published about the high cost of the negative emotions. Cancer, in particular, has been connected to intensive states of grief or anger or fear. It makes little sense to suppose that emotions exact only penalties and confer no benefits. At any rate, long before my own serious illness, I became convinced that creativity, the will to live, hope, faith, and love have biochemical significance and contribute strongly to healing and to well-being. The positive emotions are life-giving experiences.

Scientific research has established the existence of endorphins in the human brain—a substance very much like morphine in its molecular structure and effects. It is the body's own anesthesia and a relaxant and helps human beings to sustain pain. Exactly how the endorphins are activated and released into the bloodstream is not yet fully known. Nor is it known whether they might be activated by the positive emotions. But enough research has been done to indicate that those individuals with determination to overcome an illness tend to have a greater tolerance to severe pain than those who are morbidly apprehensive. Chinese medical scientists contend that the highly successful use of acupuncture instead of anesthetic is made possible because the insertion of needles in the "meridians" of the body activates the endorphins.

In any case, the human mind has a role to play in the control of pain, just as it has a key role in combating illness. We need look no further than the phenomenon of the placebo to recognize that, both on the conscious and subconscious level, the mind can order the body to react or respond in certain ways. Such response involves body chemistry and not just psychological reactions.

In the first chapter, I wrote about the ability of laughter to reduce the inflammation in my joints, confirmed by a reduction in the sedimentation rate—both sustained and cumulative. Did this mean that laughter stimulated the endorphins? An interesting experiment in this direction was undertaken by a Japanese doctor in Tokyo, who incorporated laughter into the treatment of tuberculous patients. The account of the experiment said that he was able to demonstrate to his own satisfaction that laughter was therapeutic and figured in the improvement of his patients.

Other and more comprehensive research studies and experiments will be designed. As a result we will learn a great deal more than we know about the role of the positive emotions and of creativity and of the will to live. Before long, medical researchers may discover that the human brain has a natural drive to sustain the life process and to potentiate the entire body in the fight against pain and disease. When that knowledge is developed, the art and practice of medicine will ascend to a new and higher plateau.

# 4

## Pain Is Not
## the Ultimate Enemy

Americans are probably the most pain-conscious people on the face of the earth. For years we have had it drummed into us—in print, on radio, over television, in everyday conversation—that any hint of pain is to be banished as though it were the ultimate evil. As a result, we are becoming a nation of pill-grabbers and hypochondriacs, escalating the slightest ache into a searing ordeal.

We know very little about pain and what we don't know makes it hurt all the more. Indeed, no form of illiteracy in the United States is so widespread or costly as ignorance about pain—what it is, what causes it, how to deal with it without panic. Almost everyone can rattle off the names of at least a dozen drugs that can deaden pain from every conceivable cause—all the way from headaches to hemorrhoids. There is far less knowledge about the fact that about 90 percent of pain is self-limiting, that it is not always an indication of poor health, and that, most frequently, it is the result of tension, stress, worry, idleness, boredom, frustration, suppressed rage, insufficient sleep, overeating, poorly balanced diet, smoking, excessive drinking, inadequate exercise, stale air, or any of the other abuses encountered by the human body in modern society.

The most ignored fact of all about pain is that the best way to eliminate it is to eliminate the abuse. Instead, many people reach almost instinctively for the painkillers—aspirins, barbiturates, codeines, tranquilizers, sleeping pills, and dozens of other analgesics or desensitizing drugs.

Most doctors are profoundly troubled over the extent to which the medical profession today is taking on the trappings of a pain-killing industry. Their offices are overloaded with people who are morbidly but mistakenly convinced that something dreadful is about to happen to them. It is all too evident that the campaign to get people to run to a doctor at the first sign of pain has boomeranged. Physicians find it difficult to give adequate attention to patients genuinely in need of expert diagnosis and treatment because their time is soaked up by people who have nothing wrong with them except a temporary indisposition or a psychogenic ache.

Patients tend to feel indignant and insulted if the physician tells them he can find no organic cause for the pain. They tend to interpret the term "psychogenic" to mean that they are complaining of nonexistent symptoms. They need to be educated about the fact that many forms of pain have no underlying physical cause but are the result, as mentioned earlier, of tension, stress, or hostile factors in the general environment. Sometimes a pain may be a manifestation of "conversion hysteria," as mentioned earlier, the name given by Jean Charcot to physical symptoms that have their origins in emotional disturbances.

Obviously, it is folly for an individual to ignore symptoms that could be a warning of a potentially serious illness. Some people are so terrified of getting bad news from a doctor that they allow their malaise to worsen, sometimes past the point of no return. Total neglect is not the answer to hypochondria. The only answer has to be increased education about the way the human body works, so that more people will be able to steer an intelligent course between promiscuous pill-popping and irresponsible disregard of genuine symptoms.

Of all forms of pain, none is more important for the individual to understand than the "threshold" variety. Almost everyone has a telltale ache that is triggered whenever tension or fatigue reaches a certain point. It can take the form of a migraine-type headache or a squeezing pain deep in the abdomen or cramps or a pain in the lower back or even pain in the joints. The individual who has learned how to make the correlation between such threshold pains and their cause doesn't panic when they occur; he or she does something about relieving the stress and tension. Then, if the pain persists despite the absence of apparent cause, the individual will telephone the doctor.

If ignorance about the nature of pain is widespread, ignorance about the way pain-killing drugs work is even more so. What is not generally understood is that many of the vaunted pain-killing drugs conceal the pain without correcting the underlying condition. They deaden the mechanism in the body that alerts the brain to the fact that something may be wrong. The body can pay a high price for suppression of pain without regard to its basic cause.

Professional athletes are sometimes severely disadvantaged by trainers whose job it is to keep them in action. The more famous the athlete, the greater the risk that he or she may be subjected to extreme medical measures when injury strikes. The star baseball pitcher whose arm is sore because of a torn muscle or tissue damage may need sustained rest more than anything else. But his team is battling for a place in the World Series; so the trainer or team doctor, called upon to work his magic, reaches for a strong dose of butazolidine or other powerful pain suppressants. Presto, the pain disappears! The pitcher takes his place on the mound and does superbly. That could be the last game, however, in which he is able to throw a ball with full strength. The drugs didn't repair the torn muscle or cause the damaged tissue to heal. What they did was to mask the pain, enabling the pitcher to throw hard, further damaging the torn muscle. Little wonder that so many star athletes are cut down in their prime, more the victims of overzealous treatment of their injuries than of the injuries themselves.

The king of all painkillers, of course, is aspirin. The U. S. Food and Drug Administration permits aspirin to be sold without prescription, but the drug, contrary to popular belief, can be dangerous and, in sustained doses, potentially lethal. Aspirin is self-administered by more people than any other drug in the world. Some people are aspirin-poppers, taking ten or more a day. What they don't know is that the smallest dose can cause internal bleeding. Even more serious perhaps is the fact that aspirin is antagonistic to collagen, which has a key role in the formation of connective tissue. Since many forms of arthritis involve disintegration of the connective tissue, the steady use of aspirin can actually intensify the underlying arthritic condition.

The reason why aspirin is prescribed so widely for arthritic patients is that it has an antiinflammatory effect, apart from its pain-deadening characteristics. In recent years, however, medical researchers have suggested that the antiinflammatory value of aspirin may be offset by the harm it causes to the body's vital chemistry. Doctors J. Hirsh, D. Street, J.F. Cade, and H. Amy, in the March 1973 issue of the professional journal *Blood,* showed that aspirin impedes the interaction between "platelet release" and connective tissue. In the *Annals of Rheumatic Diseases,* also in March 1973, Dr. P.N. Sperryn reported a significant blood loss in patients who were on heavy daily doses of aspirin. (It is not unusual for patients suffering from serious rheumatoid arthritis to take as many as twenty-four aspirin tablets a day.)

Again, I call attention to the article in the May 8, 1971 issue of *Lancet,* the English medical journal. Dr. M. A. Sahud and Dr. R. J. Cohen stated that the systematic use of aspirin by rheumatoid patients produces abnormally low plasma-ascorbic-acid levels. The authors reported that aspirin blocks the "uptake of ascorbic acid into the blood platelets." Since vitamin C is essential in collagen formation, its depletion by aspirin would seem to run directly counter to the body's need to combat connective tissue breakdown in arthritic conditions. The *Lancet* article concludes that, at the very least, ascorbic acid should be administered along with aspirin to counteract its harmful effects.

Aspirin is not the only pain-killing drug, of course, that is known to have dangerous side effects. Dr. Daphne A. Roe, of Cornell University, at a medical meeting in New York City in 1974, presented startling evidence of a wide range of hazards associated with sedatives and other pain suppressants. Some of these drugs seriously interfere with the ability of the body to metabolize food properly, producing malnutrition. In some instances, there is also the danger of bone-marrow depression, interfering with the ability of the body to replenish its blood supply.

Pain-killing drugs are among the greatest advances in the history of medicine. Properly used, they can be a boon in alleviating suffering and in treating disease.

But their indiscriminate and promiscuous use is making psychological cripples and chronic ailers out of millions of people. The unremitting barrage of advertising for pain-killing drugs, especially over television, has set the stage for a mass anxiety neurosis. Almost from the moment children are old enough to sit upright in front of a television screen, they are being indoctrinated into the hypochondriac's clamorous and morbid world. Little wonder so many people fear pain more than death itself.

It might be a good idea if concerned physicians and educators could get together to make knowledge about pain an important part of the regular school curriculum. As for the populace at large, perhaps some of the same techniques used by public-service agencies to make people cancer-conscious can be used to counteract the growing terror of pain and illness in general. People ought to know that nothing is more remarkable about the human body than its recuperative drive, given a modicum of respect. If our broadcasting stations cannot provide equal time for responses to the pain-killing advertisements, they might at least set aside a few minutes each day for common-sense remarks on the subject of pain. As for the Food and Drug Administration, it might be interesting to know why an agency that has so energetically warned the American people against taking vitamins without prescriptions is doing so little to control over-the-counter sales each year of billions of pain-killing pills, some of which can do more harm than the pain they are supposed to suppress.

* * *

If an account is ever written about the attempts of the medical profession to understand pain, the name of Paul Brand may have an honored place. Dr. Brand has worked with lepers for most of his medical career. He is an English orthopedic surgeon, recognized throughout world medical circles for his work in restoring crippled or paralyzed hands to productive use. His principal work at Medical College at Vellore, India, was as director of orthopedic surgery.

Paul Brand went to Vellore as a young man in 1947. His wife, also a surgeon, joined him at Vellore a year later. Together, they constituted one of the most remarkable husband-and-wife medical teams in the world. Paul Brand restored to thousands of lepers the use of their hands and arms. Margaret Brand saved thousands of lepers from blindness. Both of them taught at the medical college, undertook important research, and worked at the hospital and in field clinics.

Paul Brand's main purpose in coming to the Christian Medical College and Hospital at Vellore was to see whether he might be able to apply his highly developed skills in reconstructive surgery to the special problems of lepers. Commonly, lepers' fingers tend to "claw" or partially close up because of the paralysis of vital nerves controlling the muscles of the hand. Brand wanted to try to reactivate the fingers by connecting them to healthy nerve impulses in the leper's forearm. This would require, of course, reeducating the patient so that his brain could transmit orders to the lower forearm instead of the hand for activating the fingers.

He wasn't at Vellore very long, however, before he realized he couldn't confine himself to problems caused by the clawish hands of lepers. He would have to deal with the total problem of leprosy—what it was, how it took hold in the human body, how it might be combated. He immersed himself in research. The more he learned, the greater was his awareness that most of the attitudes toward leprosy he had carried with him to Vellore were outmoded to the point of being medieval. He became determined to pit the scientific method against the old mysteries of leprosy.

He was to discover that the prevailing ideas about "leprous tissue" were mistaken. Wrong, too, was the notion that missing toes or fingers or atrophy of the nose were direct products or manifestations of the disease. Most significant of all perhaps was his awareness that leprosy was a disease of painlessness.

As head of the research section, Paul Brand first needed to find out as much as he could about tissue from the affected parts of lepers. Medicine had long known that leprosy was produced by a bacillus somewhat similar to the organism that causes tuberculosis. This discovery had been made by Gerhard Henrik Hansen almost a century and a half ago; the term "Hansen's disease" became synonymous with leprosy. As in the case of tuberculosis, the *bacillus leprae* produced tubercles. The leprosy tubercles varied in size

97

from a small pea to a large olive. They appeared on the face, ears, and bodily extremities. It was commonly thought that the bacillus was responsible in some way for the sloughing-off of fingers and toes, and even of hands and feet. Yet very little had been done in actual tissue research. Was there anything in the flesh of finger stumps or toes that differentiated this tissue from healthy cells? Was the *bacillus leprae* an active agent in the atrophy? Dr. Brand put the pathologists to work. Through research, they came up with the startling finding that there was no difference between healthy tissue and the tissue of a leper's fingers or toes.

One point, however, was scientifically certain: the *bacillus leprae* killed nerve endings. This meant that the delicate sense of touch was missing or seriously injured. But the flesh itself, Dr. Brand ascertained, was otherwise indistinguishable from normal tissue.

As is often the case in medical research, some of Paul Brand's most important discoveries about leprosy came about not as the result of systematic pursuit but through accident. Soon after arriving in Vellore he observed the prodigious strength in lepers' hands. Even a casual handshake with a leper was like putting one's fingers in a vise. Was this because something in the disease released manual strength not known to healthy people?

The answer came one day when Paul Brand was unable to turn a key in a large rusty lock. A leprous boy of twelve observed Dr. Brand's difficulty and asked to help. Dr. Brand was astonished at the ease with which the youngster turned the key. He examined the boy's thumb and forefinger of the right hand. The key had cut the flesh to the bone. The boy had been completely unaware of what was happening to his fingers while turning the key.

Dr. Brand had his answer at once. The desensitized nerve endings had made it possible for the child to keep turning the key long past the point where a healthy person would have found it painful to continue. Healthy people possess strength they never use precisely because resistant pressure causes pain. A leper's hands are not more powerful, he reasoned; they just lack the mechanism of pain to tell them when to stop applying pressure. In this way serious damage could be done to flesh and bone.

Was it possible, Dr. Brand asked himself, that the reason lepers lost fingers and toes was not because of leprosy itself but because they were insensitive to injury? In short, could a person be unaware that, in the ordinary course of a day's activity, he might be subjecting his body to serious physical damage? Paul Brand analyzed all the things he himself did in the course of a day—turning faucets and doorknobs, operating levers, dislodging or pulling or pushing things, using utensils of all kinds. In most of these actions, pressure was required. And the amount of pressure was determined both by the resistance of the object and the ability of his fingers and hands to tolerate stress. Lacking the sensitivity, he knew, he would continue to exert pressure even though damage to his hands might be incurred in the process.

He observed lepers as they went about their daily

tasks and was convinced he was correct. He began to educate lepers in stress tolerance; he designed special gloves to protect their hands; and he set up daily examinations so that injuries would not lead to ulceration and to disfigurement, as had previously occurred. Almost miraculously, the incidence of new injuries was sharply reduced. Lepers became more productive. Paul Brand began to feel he was making basic progress.

Some mysteries, however, persisted. How to account for the continuing disappearance of fingers, in part or whole? Why was it that parts of fingers would vanish from one day to the next. Were they knocked off? There was nothing to indicate that bones of lepers were any more brittle than the bones of normal people. If a leper cut off a finger while using a saw, or if a finger were somehow broken off, it should be possible to produce the missing digit. But no one ever found a finger after it had been lost. Why?

Paul Brand thought about the problem. Then, suddenly, the answer flashed through his mind. It had to be rats. And it would happen at night, while the lepers were asleep. Since the hands of lepers were desensitized, they wouldn't know they were being attacked and so would put up no resistance.

Paul Brand set up observation posts at night in the huts and wards. It was just as he had thought. The rats climbed the beds of lepers, sniffed carefully, and, when they encountered no resistance, went to work on fingers and toes. The fingers hadn't been dropping off; they were being eaten. This didn't mean that all "lost" fingers had disappeared in this way. They could be knocked off through accidents and then carried away by rats or other animals before the loss would be observed. But a major cause of the disappearance had now been identified.

Paul Brand and his staff went to work, mounting a double-pronged attack against the invaders. The program for rodent control was stepped up many times. Barriers were built around the legs of beds. The beds themselves were raised. The results were immediately apparent. There was a sharp drop in the disappearance of fingers and toes.

All this time, Paul Brand kept up his main work— reconstructing hands, rerouting muscles, straightening out fingers. Where fingers were shortened or absent, the remaining digits had to be made fully operative. Thousands of lepers were restored to manual productivity.

One of the grim but familiar marks of many lepers is the apparent decay of their noses. What caused the shrinkage? It was highly unlikely that the nose suffered from the kind of persistent injury that frequently affected the desensitized hands and feet. What about rats? This, too, seemed unlikely. Enough sensitivity existed in a leper's face, especially around the mouth, to argue strongly against the notion of rodent assault.

As Paul Brand pursued the riddle, he became convinced that neither injuries nor rats were involved. Finally, he found his answer in his research on the effect of *bacillus leprae* on the delicate membranes inside the nose. These membranes would contract

ANATOMY OF AN ILLNESS

severely in lepers. This meant that the connecting cartilage would be yanked inward. What was happening, therefore, was not decay or loss of nasal structure through injury. The nose was being drawn into the head.

It was a startling discovery, running counter to medical ideas that had lasted for centuries. Could Brand prove it? The best way of proceeding, he felt, was by surgery that would push the nose back into the face. He therefore reconstructed the nose from the inside. It was a revolutionary approach.

He knew that the operation couldn't work in all cases. Where the leprosy was so far advanced that membrane shrinkage left little to work with, it was doubtful that the operation would be successful. But there was a good chance that, in those cases where the disease could be arrested and where the shrinkage was not extreme, noses could be pushed back into place.

The theory worked. As a result, the nose restorative operation developed at Vellore has been used for the benefit of large numbers of lepers at hospitals throughout the world.

Next, blindness. Of all the afflictions of leprosy, perhaps none is more serious or characteristic than blindness. Here, too, it had been assumed for many centuries that loss of sight was a specific manifestation of advanced leprosy. At Vellore, this assumption was severely questioned. Intensive study of the disease convinced Paul Brand and his fellow researchers that blindness was not a direct product of leprosy but a by-product. A serious vitamin A deficiency, for example, could be a major contributing cause of cataracts and consequent blindness. Where cataracts were already formed, it was possible to remove them by surgery.

It was in this field that Dr. Margaret Brand became especially active and effective. On some days she would perform as many as a hundred cataract operations. This number would seem high to the point of absurdity to many European and American eye surgeons for whom twelve such operations in a single day would be considered formidable. But the eye surgeons at Vellore have to contend with literally thousands of people waiting in line to be saved from blindness. They often work fourteen to sixteen hours a day, using techniques that facilitate rapid surgery.

Dr. Margaret Brand was part of a medical and surgical field team that would make regular rounds among villages far removed from the hospital. Surgical tents would be set up. Electricity would be supplied by power take-off devices from the jeep motors.

Cataracts, however, were not the whole story in blindness among lepers. Many lepers at Vellore didn't suffer from cataracts, yet were losing their sight from eye ulcerations. Did the *bacillus leprae* produce the infection and the resultant ulcerations and blindness? Or, as in the case of fingers and toes, was the loss of function a by-product in which other causes had to be identified and eliminated.

The latter line of reasoning proved to be fruitful. Human eyes are constantly exposed to all sorts of irritations from dust and dirt in the air. The eyes deal with these invasions almost without a person being aware of the process. Thousands of times a day the eyelids close and open, washing the surface of the eye with soothing saline fluid released by the tear ducts.

Paul Brand and his colleagues believed this washing process didn't take place in lepers because there was a loss of sensation on the eye surface caused by the atrophy of nerve endings. This hypothesis was easily and readily confirmed. They observed the eyes of lepers when subjected to ordinary irritations. There was, as they had suspected, no batting of the eyelids; therefore, there could be no washing process. The big problem, then, was to get the eyelids working again.

Why not educate lepers to make a conscious effort to bat their eyes? There being no impairment of a leper's ability to close his eyes at will, it ought to be possible to train lepers to be diligent in this respect. But experiments quickly demonstrated the disadvantages of this approach. Unless a leper concentrated on the matter constantly, it wouldn't work. And if he did concentrate, he could think of almost nothing else. No; what was needed was a way of causing eyelid action that would clean the eyes automatically.

In the case of fingers or toes, it was possible to educate lepers in stress tolerances and to give them protective gloves or shoes. How to keep dirt and foreign objects from getting into the eye? Eye goggles might be one answer but they were not airtight, were cumbersome, would fog up because of the high humidity, and were too easily lost. Something more basic would have to be found.

The answer, again, was found in reconstructive surgery. Paul Brand and his team devised a way of hooking up the muscles of the jaw to the eyelid. Every time a leper opened his mouth the new facial muscles would pull the eyelids and cause them to close, thus washing the eyeball. In this way, a leper could literally talk and eat his way out of oncoming blindness. Countless numbers of lepers have their sight today because of this ingenious use of surgery in facilitating the use of nature's mechanism to get rid of dirt and dust in the eyes.

* * *

Gradually, as the result of research at Vellore and other leper centers throughout the world, the terrible black superstition about leprosy is receding. Contrary to popular impressions, it is not highly contagious. In fact, it is virtually impossible to transmit leprosy to a healthy person. As with tuberculosis, of course, persons in weakened conditions are vulnerable in varying degrees. The disease is not hereditary; again, however, as with other diseases, increased susceptibility can be passed along from parent to child.

Basically, leprosy is the product of filth, poverty, and malnutrition. It is not, as is generally supposed, a disease of the tropics and subtropics. It can exist wherever unsanitary conditions, hunger, or poorly balanced diet exist. It has existed in countries as far north as Iceland. Scarcely a country in the world has been untouched by it. But the important thing is that it is eradicable, and its victims can be cured or appreciably helped and rehabilitated. And it can once and for all be rescued from the general ignorance and associated superstitions assigned to it over the ages.

Medical researchers have given high recognition to Dr. Brand and his colleagues for their new insights into the nature of leprosy, but even greater accolades within the profession have come his way because of his work in rehabilitative surgery. He has been able to transform hands, long clawed and rigid because of nerve atrophy brought on by leprosy or other causes, into functioning mechanisms. Almost legendary in India is the case of a lawyer on whom he operated. For many years, the lawyer had been at a disadvantage in court. His gestures, so essential a part of the dramatic courtroom manner, were actually a liability; judge and jury were distracted by the hideously deformed and frozen hand. Then one day the lawyer raised his hand to emphasize a point. The hand was supple; the fingers moved, the gesture was appropriate. Paul Brand had operated on the hand, hooking up muscle and nerve connections to the forearm, then educating the patient to retrain his command impulses.

Paul Brand and his staff have performed thousands of similar operations on patients at Vellore. But they have also gone far beyond surgery into what they consider an even more vital phase of the total treatment. This is psychological rehabilitation. A man who, as a leper, has been a beggar for twenty years is not considered to be fully treated at Vellore until he is mentally and physically prepared to be a useful and proud citizen in his society. At Vellore, handicapped patients are given the kind of training that will enable them to be as self-supporting as possible. They gain a respect for the limitless potentialities and adaptabilities of the human organism. They learn that even as little as a 10 percent mobility can be made to yield a high return in terms of effective productivity. And, in the Emersonian sense, self-reliance creates self-respect.

It is not necessary, of course, to provide any precise assessment of the relative importance of the three main phases of Paul Brand's work—taking the black curse and superstition out of leprosy, reconstructive surgery, and personal and psychological rehabilitation. All are important; all are interrelated. But one aspect of his work may perhaps be more evocative and compelling than any of the others. He is a doctor who, if he could, would move heaven and earth just to return the gift of pain to people who do not have it. For pain is both the warning system and the protective mechanism that enables an individual to defend the integrity of his body. Its signals may not always be readily intelligible but at least they are there. And the individual can mobilize his response.

# 5

## Holistic Health
## and Healing

One of the results of the article in the *New England Journal of Medicine* was that I had opportunities to observe the holistic health movement at first hand. Leaders of the movement were good enough to say that I had had a holistic experience and that they hoped I might come to their meetings to talk about that experience as a way of reinforcing the beliefs of its members.

My problem, however, was that I had said as much as I thought I ought to say about the illness itself. Besides, I was aware of the tendency of a few advocates in the movement to juxtapose themselves against the entire medical profession, and I couldn't sympathize with this approach. While I agreed with the prime tenets of the holistic movement, I saw a need to build bridges across the gap that for so long had separated the physician and the public. Moreover, what to me was most impressive, as I explain more fully in the next chapter, about the thousands of letters I received from doctors in response to the *NEJM* piece, was the sense of an important new mood in American medicine. I believed that the holistic movement would be gratified by the fast-growing evidence that many doctors were attempting to diagnose and treat the patient in the context of all the factors—work, nutrition, family, personality, emotions, environment—that figure in illness or breakdown.

In accepting invitations to speak or participate at these meetings, therefore, I sought—and received—permission to talk about the need to avoid a wall of separation between patients and physicians. It was true that the medical profession had allowed itself to become overly mystifying, even authoritarian, in its general relationships with the community-at-large. But there were genuine signs of a desire to inform and educate and not superimpose. Patients were being encouraged by their physicians to know as much as possible about issues involving their health. What was in the making, it seemed to me, was an expanding dialogue between the public and the profession on the proper division of responsibility between the two.

Such a dialogue, I felt certain, would impress physicians with the seriousness and soundness of intent of millions of people who believe that the primary role of the doctor is to help people to prevent illness, and not just to overcome it. And people in the movement, I felt equally convinced, would be impressed by the large number of doctors whose philosophy and practice were based on the idea that the mind and body are a single organism, and that the treatment of either one should not be undertaken without respect for the totality.

Great medical teachers have always impressed upon their students the need to make a careful assessment of everything that may interact in the cause and course of a disease. Hippocrates, the first major historical name in medicine, was both a theoretician and a practitioner. He tried to close existing gaps between the understanding of disease and its treatment. He was quintessentially holistic when he insisted that it is natural for the human body to heal itself, and that this process can generally take place even without the intervention of a physician *(vis medicatrix naturae)*. He believed that the essential function of the physician— here again Hippocrates was being nothing if not holistic—was to avoid any treatment that might interfere with the healing process or that might do harm *(primum non nocere)*.

Hippocrates put his emphasis on the systematic organization and application of knowledge. He was troubled by the fact that a great deal of dogma and superstition were being dressed up as carefully authenticated principles in the practice of medicine. Lawrence J. Henderson, widely admired among modern teachers of medicine, described the essence

111

of these principles in one of his famous Harvard lectures.

Hippocrates was no casual ordinary observer, Henderson wrote, but a physician whose "skill depended upon both native capacity and long practice. . . . His success was great, and the whole history of science goes far to support the view that such a methodical procedure is a necessary step in the development of a science that deals with similarly complex and various phenomena."

This holistic principle has been restated many times as a basic guideline for sound medical practice. A half-century ago, Arturo Castiglioni, in his *A History of Medicine,* wrote that "the physician above all should keep in mind the welfare of the patient, his constantly changing state, not only in the visible signs of his illness but also in his state of mind, which must necessarily be an important factor in the success of the treatment. One would be blind not to recognize that before and even after the advent of modern scientific medicine there were great and able healers of the sick who were not men of science, but who had the ability to reassure the patient and thus favorably to influence the course of the illness. It is also obvious that there have been excellent scientists who were very mediocre practitioners. Thus history teaches that any division of the science and art of medicine is necessarily harmful to practice."

If holistic concepts are not new, how are we to account for the extraordinary new popular interest and its development into a national and indeed a worldwide movement? At least half a dozen factors are involved.

Ever since the dangers of thalidomide for pregnant women were discovered, many thousands of people have become aware that modern drugs are not to be regarded solely in a life-saving role; they can be powerfully dangerous, even when taken as directed by the physician. Antibiotics made their appearance as miracle drugs; they were able to destroy potent microorganisms beyond the reach of other medications. But bacteria became inured and resistant to the antibiotics, requiring ever more powerful forms of antibiotic killers. This in turn made the human body increasingly vulnerable to the harmful effects of the antibiotics. The chain reaction was costly and destructive. So the physician had to weigh carefully the relative dangers and benefits. The same was true of steroid drugs. The dramatic and almost instantaneous improvements brought about by the cortisones had to be balanced off against disturbances to the endocrine system.

There were other new drugs, more effective than ever before in preventing or combating hypertension, or in regulating the human heartbeat, or in restoring sluggish organs, or in combating unusual growths—all of them powerfully effective but each imposing penalties or risks. These dangers were often as great as, and sometimes greater than, the benefits; their use was therefore brought into serious question.

The public's awareness of these dangers rose very sharply in the 1960s and 1970s, as consumer consciousness expanded into the health field. The result was a growing distrust not just of the highly sophisticated new drugs but of almost all medications in general. People became attracted to the emphasis of holistic medicine on eliminating basic causes of breakdown and illness rather than on the use of hazardous drugs. It was felt that doctors had a tendency to overmedicate and to fail to maintain the necessary vigilance over patients who continued to take potent drugs long past the point where their use was indicated—often resulting in health problems even more severe than the ones for which the medication was originally prescribed. People tended to forget that much of the pressure on doctors to prescribe the exotic new drugs came from the public itself.

In any case, the reaction against drugs became an important part of the appeal of holistic medicine.

Inevitably, the distrust of powerful medication figured in the surging new emphasis on proper nutrition, which was seen both as a precondition of good health and as a substitute for drugs in the treatment of many illnesses. Books on nutrition found an eager audience. One author, Adelle Davis, produced a succession of books on nutrition that for a half-dozen years or more outsold everything between covers except the Bible. Carlton Fredericks's radio program on nutrition found an audience in the millions. One of the fastest-growing magazines in America was *Prevention*, which put its dominant emphasis on health through proper nutrition, and which carried reports of the growth of the holistic health movement.

The public became aware, as the result of the

White House Conference on Food, Nutrition, and Health in 1969, and through the growing literature of protest against drugs, that medical schools failed to teach nutrition or at least to accord it the same importance in their curricula as physiology, pathology, pharmacology, anatomy, biochemistry, and so on. Actually, nutrition was not being ignored or bypassed, but was taught as an integral part of other subjects. Even so, the fact that it had no standing of its own in most medical schools ran counter to the public's conviction that nutrition was at the very top of factors affecting health. And the more some doctors tried to combat this view—generally by asserting that the average food market shopping basket provided everything needed for a balanced diet—the more convinced people became that doctors were opposed to them on nutritional matters. The fact that so few doctors questioned their patients in detail about their food habits provided yet additional evidence on this point.

At the same time, the general practitioner has had no way of keeping up with fast-developing new knowledge, let alone the vast array of new technology and techniques. Even as they made allowances for these facts, however, the public felt uncomfortable about the extent to which specialization was changing medical practice. People saw a contradiction between the traditional view of the doctor as a reassuring father figure who took care of all their medical needs, and the pluralization of the doctor-patient relationship brought about by specialists who presided over separate parts of their anatomy. Holistic medicine has

ANATOMY OF AN ILLNESS

tried to counteract this trend by putting emphasis on
the integrating factors.

The emergence of specialists was connected to the
burgeoning new medical technology, giving many
people the impression that the doctor was an auxiliary
of the machine. Patients found it difficult to accept the
new impersonalization produced by the new technology. Moreover, the machines pronounced verdicts
with a finality that seemed to run counter to one of the
oldest rules of medical diagnosis: always allow for the
fact that certain individuals may have all the signs and
symptoms of a particular disease, yet may be atypical
or even completely free of that disease. In any case,
holistic medicine put its emphasis on human contact
and human warmth, regarding medical technology as
generally cold and unappealing.

There has been a need in the nation for increasing the number of doctors who would serve rural
areas or work in inner-city community clinics; yet
the large majority of medical school graduates have
been attracted to specialized practice in the big cities.
Doctors are criticized for seeking the big incomes
that metropolitan centers make possible, but this
criticism doesn't take into account the fact that a
large number of medical school graduates have to
pay off tuition debts that often exceed $50,000. It
would be a mistake to doubt the sincerity of students
who say they would be far more disposed to work in
country clinics if their massive educational debts
were not hanging over them. Whatever the justification, the fact remains that people who need doctors

the most are least able to get to them, or, if they do manage to get to them, are least able to meet the general level of fees in private practice.

The rapid rise in the educational level of Americans was reflected in the ability of many people to inform themselves to a far greater extent than ever before about health matters. Many millions of Americans got into the habit of following medical developments. In their own relationships with physicians they no longer were disposed to accept medical decisions unquestioningly. They tended to evaluate doctors according to the willingness of the physician to enter into a mutually respectful dialogue with them.

Enough verifiable data have appeared about the ability of the human mind to play a major role in overcoming illness to make this entire field enormously attractive to laymen. It is manifestly true that interest in these matters outruns systematic knowledge; many people eagerly snatch at new findings or speculations having to do with the reach of the mind. And they are disappointed when they discover that their doctors are not equally well-informed or excited about such developments and prospects. With each new popular book on the potentialities of the human mind or on its influence over the autonomic nervous system, the gap has widened between the public and the medical profession. Not all doctors, of course, are disdainful of the new trends. The biochemical manifestations of mental powers are being well-documented. Competent observers have written about yogis in India, for example, who were trained to slow down their pulse to a few beats per minute, or who can order their skin to resist burning from hot surfaces. I myself have witnessed such demonstrations in India, so I know them to be true. But systematic scrutiny of such phenomena has lagged behind popular interest, the result being that the entire field has been colored by guesswork and extraordinary claims. Out of it all, however, has emerged the undeniable evidence that the human mind can be trained to play an important part both in preventing disease and in overcoming it when it occurs. The entire biofeedback movement has gained in stature as the result of such new research. In any case, many thousands of Americans are pressing for greater emphasis—by the medical profession—on mind-body interactions and the attack on illness.

To be sure, these are not the only elements involved in the burgeoning growth of the holistic health movement. But they constitute both the main structural props and the rallying points for the growing interest of the educated public. Underlying these ideas, of course, are the traditional essentials of health that have always had a strong place in medical canons —proper nutrition, adequate exercise, enough sleep, good air, moderation in personal habits, and so on.

* * *

At the various holistic health conferences I attended, I became aware of a troubling contradiction. A movement based on the concept of wholeness was itself becoming unwhole. Two dozen or more schools or approaches of varying validity, not all of them compatible and some of them competitive, were crowding the center of the holistic stage. Some conferences on holistic health seemed more like a congeries of exhibits and separate theories than the occasion for articulating a cohesive philosophy. Generally included were exhibits or presentations from acupuncture, astrology, graphology, numerology, clairvoyance, biofeedback, homeopathy, naturopathy, nutrition, iridology, pyramidology, psychic surgery, yoga, faith healing, vitamin therapy, apricot kernel therapy, touch encounters, chiropractic, self-massage, negative ionization, and psychocalisthenics, among others.

The inclusion of all these approaches in the same paragraph creates an impression that acupuncture, for example, is on the same level as astrology in the treatment of illness. The same is true when they come together in a conference or exhibit hall. I recognize that many people believe that astrology is a valid guide to treatment of serious illness. I respect their right to that opinion, but I would not want to take the responsibility for advising anyone who is seriously ill to forego the soundest medical advice obtainable. In any case, it is difficult to think of a unifying principle that can tie together nutrition and graphology in a systematic approach to good health. Indeed, the danger of fragmentation and general diffusion in such a coupling is all too real. The parts seem to be at odds with a movement based on the need for an integrated approach to health. One of the dangers is that the movement tends to take on the character of the least workable and reputable of the contending parts.

While it is reasonable, therefore, to expect the physician to take the concept of holistic health seriously, it is unreasonable to expect him to embrace approaches which lack systematic and sustained verifiable data. As evidence is developed, however, it is reasonable to expect the physician to examine it carefully and fully.

Similarly, it is reasonable to expect the physician to maintain an open mind about new developments in diagnosis and treatment even though they may not seem to be in harmony with his own training and experience. But it is not reasonable to expect him to proceed with any treatment in the absence of adequate clinical evidence that it is safe and efficacious. No responsible doctor will experiment with his patients.

It is reasonable to expect the physician to have respect for the powers of mind in overcoming disease, especially in view of the laboratory and clinical evidence that human biochemistry is affected by will-power or emotional states. But it is unreasonable to expect him to give those approaches a monopoly status in his care of patients and to abandon other methods he knows to be efficacious in varying degrees.

It is reasonable to expect the doctor to recognize that science may not have all the answers to problems of health and healing. But it is not reasonable to expect him to give up the scientific method in treating his patients. The most important thing about science is the scientific method—a way of thinking systematically, a way of assembling evidence and appraising it, a way of conducting experiments so as to predict accurately what will happen under given circumstances, a way of ascertaining and recognizing one's own errors, a way of finding the fallacies in long-held ideas. Science itself is constantly changing, largely as the result of the scientific method. It is unreasonable, therefore, to expect the doctor to depart from this method no matter how great the compulsion or persuasion.

It is reasonable to expect the doctor to accord nutrition a high place in the understanding and treatment of illness. It is equally reasonable to expect him to listen to his patient's own developed interest in the subject, even though the doctor may see logical and factual gaps in the patient's articulation. It would be a serious mistake for the physician to allow his superior knowledge of health care in general to lead him to believe that there are no particulars in which laymen may be better informed. The case for good nutrition is exactly the same as the case for good medicine. If medication can make a difference in the internal functions of a human being, so can food. It is a serious error to suppose, therefore, that medication can accomplish a desired purpose despite everything else that is taken into the human body, or that the right foods cannot be used effectively to fight disease, whether in combination with medication or without it, depending on the nature of the problem. In any case, it is reasonable to expect the physician to take a complete nutritional profile of a patient as an essential part of any examination workup.

It is unreasonable, however, to expect a physician

to believe that the right foods, however essential, are all that is required to cure any disease. The doctor would be irresponsible if he did not use all the means at his command in cases requiring heroic intervention. To the extent that proper foods are required, they should be fully employed; to the extent that the science of medicine should be fully invoked, the doctor should not be expected to hold back. If a patient has had an attack of bacterial endocarditis, for example, prompt medicinal treatment can represent the difference between life and death. Good food can play an important role in strengthening the heart, but in an emergency situation, it would be folly to abstain from drastic medicinal treatment, taking into account the remarkably high percentage of cases that have recovered swiftly when so treated.

It is reasonable to expect the physician to accept the need for vitamin supplementation where people are under stress or are subjected to environmental strains and hazards. The notion that the average diet supplies all the proper vitamin levels is not very meaningful; the use of the word "average" in such matters is arbitrary and unscientific. Some lifestyles produce a chronic vitamin imbalance. It is possible that more patients would go to doctors for advice concerning these matters if they did not have the feeling that doctors regard vitamin deficiencies as nonsense. Such deficiencies are all too real, especially as the result of the large dependence on processed foods.

It is unreasonable, however, to expect the physician to see all diseases as a manifestation of vitamin deficiency. It is equally unreasonable to expect physicians to encourage their patients to spend large sums of money on vitamins regardless of need and regardless of the possible harm that overloading might cause.

What is needed here—as it is in all matters—is a sense of balance that neither attempts to dismiss vitamins out of hand nor regards them as the only key to good health. Such a balance is possible, given attitudes of reasonableness by both physician and patient.

The holistic health movement can discover its greatest effectiveness by seeking such a balance. It would not be in the interest of the movement to regard the medical profession as the enemy. Talk of enemies does not sit well in a movement in which spiritual factors are no less vital than practical ones. Holism means healing—not just of bodies but of relationships. One of the most useful things the movement can do is to bring public and physician together in mutual respect for the ability of the human body to be fully potentiated in maintaining health and in overcoming disease. The impressive number of medical schools that are represented at various holistic health meetings around the country confirms the fact that holistic health advocates have won their main objective, which is to shift the emphasis from knowledge of the disease to knowledge of human beings in whom the disease exists.

Few things have been more encouraging for the holistic health movement than the 1978 convention of the American Medical Association. At that meeting, the nation's doctors heard talks about the dangers of overmedication and about the need for restraint in writing prescriptions in general; about the importance of psychological factors such as compassion and warmth in the treatment of the ill; about the role of good food in preventing and overcoming illness; and about ascorbic acid therapy. Linus Pauling, who only a few years ago was heavily criticized by the medical profession, made a major presentation at the convention, and provided a step-by-step account of his work with what he called "orthomolecular medicine." He seemed to have a profound impact on all those who heard him.

The auspicious prospect is that the interest of laymen can be knowledgeably applied in concert with the medical profession's own respect for the layman's responsible involvement in holistic approaches to health.

# 6

## What I Learned from Three Thousand Doctors

Following the publication in the *New England Journal of Medicine* of the first chapter of this book, I was the recipient of some three thousand letters from doctors in about a dozen countries. What was most remarkable and gratifying about these letters was the evidence of an increasingly open attitude by many doctors to new and even unconventional approaches in the treatment of serious disease. There was encouraging support in these letters for the measures that had figured in my own recovery—a well-developed will to live, laughter, and large intravenous doses of sodium ascorbate. Far from resenting the intrusion of a layman into problems of diagnosis and therapy, the doctors who wrote in response to the article warmly endorsed the idea of a patient's partnership with his physician in the search for a cure.

The letters reflected the view that one of the main functions of the doctor is to engage to the fullest the patient's own ability to mobilize the forces of mind and body in turning back disease. There was general agreement in the letters that modern medication is becoming increasingly dangerous and that, to the fullest extent, the careful physician should attempt to educate the patient away from reliance on exotic drugs. The new trend favors an understanding of the powerful recuperative and regenerative forces possessed by the human body under conditions of proper nourishment and reasonable freedom from stress.

Not all the communications came from doctors. One episode involving a layman underlines many of the key points raised by the physicians. A New York lawyer telephoned to say that his four-year-old daughter was in a coma and in critical condition in Lenox Hill Hospital. She was stricken with viral encephalitis, against which antibiotics have no record of success. It was difficult for him to accept the fact that nothing more could be done than was being done. The lawyer wanted to know whether, in the light of my own recovery from a severe collagen disease after taking large doses of ascorbic acid, the same treatment might be useful for his daughter.

I told the lawyer that it would be highly irresponsible for me, a layman like himself, to attempt to give medical advice. Moreover, there was no way of deter-

mining what part of my recovery was due to the intravenous infusion of ascorbate and what part to a full
mobilization of the salutary emotions, not excluding
laughter or a robust will to live. I suggested that the
lawyer consult his daughter's physician about the possible use of ascorbic acid.

The lawyer said he feared the child's doctor would
be scornful of anything as unsophisticated and over-
popularized as vitamin C. I then told him of the large
number of medical tracts I had received from doctors,
in response to my article, supporting the use of ascorbate in a wide range of disorders beyond the reach of
antibiotics or other medication.

In particular, I spoke of the work of Irwin Stone,
a biochemist in San Jose, who is among the country's
leading authorities on the efficacy of ascorbic acid in
the treatment of serious disease. I offered to send the
lawyer reprints of articles from medical journals
about the work of Stone and others on the functions
of ascorbate in body chemistry. What seemed especially impressive to me about these papers was the
data on the ability of ascorbate to activate and enhance
the body's own healing mechanism. I suggested that
the lawyer might wish to review this material with the
child's doctor in the event he had not already seen it.

The next day I left for a new round of the Dartmouth conferences in Latvia, U.S.S.R.—fourteen
years after the Dartmouth meeting described in the
opening chapter. While abroad, I made inquiries at
various medical centers and learned that intravenous
infusions of ascorbic acid had been effectively used in

a number of cases of viral encephalitis.

On my return to New York, I telephoned the lawyer to ask about his daughter. He said he had spoken with Irwin Stone, who told him about recent experiences in which serious cases of viral encephalitis had been reversed through large doses of ascorbate. Armed with this information and with reprints from medical journals I had sent him, the lawyer had spoken to the child's specialist, only to be rebuffed. When he had offered the materials from the professional journals, the doctor had said he didn't need to be instructed by a layman in medical matters.

The lawyer then decided on a plan of action. Several days later he asked the specialist whether the next time his child came out of the coma he might offer her some ice cream. The specialist encouraged the lawyer to do so. The lawyer bought a pound of sodium ascorbate, which is more soluble and less bitter than the ascorbic acid form. He mixed at least 10 grams of the powder into the ice cream, which he put in a thermos jug. He took the jug with him to the hospital, where he stationed himself full time. When his little girl came out of the coma, he asked whether she would like some ice cream. The reply was an enthusiastic yes. He was elated when she gobbled up most of the pint.

The next day the lawyer again gave his daughter a large portion of ice cream, enriched this time with an even stronger dose of sodium ascorbate than before. He continued the process day after day, and each day, the child would be able to spend longer periods of time out of the oxygen tent. The improvement continued steadily in the following days, during which the lawyer gave his daughter an average of 25 grams of sodium ascorbate daily. After two weeks the child was taken out of the oxygen tent altogether.

The lawyer's voice vibrated with excitement over the telephone as he told me of the child's complete recovery and the prospect of having her home again. I asked if he had informed the specialist what he had done.

"Certainly not," he replied. "Why should I make trouble for myself?"

Obviously, it is poor—and dangerous—policy for any layman to act behind a doctor's back. Yet there may be something about the specialist's attitude that warrants scrutiny. Was there a hardening of the categories that caused him to shut himself off from a serious consideration of alternatives? Was he overreacting to what he regarded as an intrusion? One of the most striking features that emerged from the letters I received from doctors is the evidence of a new respect for the ideas of nonprofessionals. "Nothing is more out of date than the notion that doctors can't learn from their patients," wrote Dr. Gerald Looney, of the Medical College of the University of Southern California. "People today are far better educated in medical matters than they were only a quarter century ago. The entire field of nutrition, for example, is one in which many patients can hold their own, to say the least, with their doctors. Maybe the new spirit of consumerism has at last reached medicine. I teach my students to listen very carefully to their patients and to concerned and informed laymen. Good medical practice begins with good listening."

One of the attractive characteristics of ascorbate is that, properly administered,* it does no harm even if it may do little good. Under these circumstances, was there any justification for the total refusal of the child's specialist to give serious consideration to the lawyer's request? Is the obligation of the doctor confined only to the patient? What about the legitimate emotional needs of those very close to the patient? The specialist's relationship with the child was limited in chronology and circumstance; the father had a lifetime commitment.

Another example of a problem arising from a doctor's dealings with a relative of a patient concerns the wife of a man dying from cancer in Boston. She telephoned to say her husband had been through the standard treatment—radiation, surgery, and chemotherapy—and she was despairing about the future. She had read that Linus Pauling, the Nobel Prize-winning chemist, had said that vitamin C is a cure for cancer. Her hopes had been raised by this prospect, and she wanted to know if, on the basis of my own experience with a supposedly irreversible illness, I thought ascorbic acid ought to be tried.

As in the case of my conversation with the lawyer, I told the woman that it would be highly improper for me to attempt to give advice. I did, however, call her

---

*The problems of improper administration are discussed later in this chapter.

attention to the fact that Dr. Pauling's conclusions were based largely on the research of Dr. Ewan Cameron, of the Vale of Leven Hospital in Loch Lomondside, Scotland. Dr. Cameron was careful not to claim that ascorbic acid was a cure for cancer. His work indicated that ascorbic acid would *prolong* the survival time of cancer victims but would not *reverse* cancer. His studies involved one hundred patients suffering from advanced malignancies who were given large doses of sodium ascorbate over a period of many weeks. The results were compared with the experiences of a thousand cancer patients of similar condition who were given no ascorbate. The average survival time of the patients in the first group was substantially longer than that of the second group. (It is important to note that "substantially" means a matter of weeks or months, and not years. While Dr. Cameron sees no evidence that ascorbic acid can expunge cancer, he believes that his work is significant in that it clearly indicates that ascorbate has cancer-retardant qualities.)

Cancer cells, Dr. Cameron says, release hyaluronidase, an enzyme that attacks intercellular cement. "Proliferation will continue as long as hyaluronidase is released; proliferation will stop when the release of hyaluronidase stops." Ascorbic acid, according to Dr. Cameron, strengthens tissue-grounding and therefore counteracts hyaluronidase activity.

Such, at least, was the gist of the material that I offered to send to the woman in Boston whose husband was dying of cancer. I emphasized that ascorbic acid could not be regarded as a proven cure for cancer or other advanced diseases. She asked whether I would be willing to discuss these matters with her husband's doctor. I told her I thought this would be inappropriate but suggested that her doctor might like to talk to my own physician, Dr. William Hitzig, who had provided full support for my decision to discontinue aspirin, butazolidin, colchicine, and sleeping pills—all of which were toxic in varying degrees—and to seek to reverse my condition through a comprehensive regimen, only one part of which was regular intravenous doses of ascorbate.

The woman telephoned two days later to say she had attempted to discuss the possible efficacy of ascorbate for her husband, only to have the doctor cut her short by chanting "quack, quack" and then describing the whole process as "b. s."

The woman and her husband decided to discontinue the doctor's services, although he had been a longtime family friend. They also decided to leave the hospital and to return home, where the atmosphere made for a less stressful environment and where a local doctor was glad to administer the sodium ascorbate.

Their course of action produced results similar to the findings reported by Dr. Cameron. The husband gained some ground. His appetite improved; so did his will to live. He succumbed to cancer after six months—four or five months later than the original prognosis. Most important, perhaps, was that he was able to spend his remaining time in congenial surroundings in the company of his wife.

Death is not the ultimate tragedy of life. The ultimate tragedy is depersonalization—dying in an alien and sterile area, separated from the spiritual nourishment that comes from being able to reach out to a loving hand, separated from a desire to experience the things that make life worth living, separated from hope.

The trend in modern medicine is to move away from the notion that it is always mandatory to hospitalize seriously ill patients. The great technological advances in electronic equipment, typified by the hospital intensive-care unit, are not without their built-in penalties. A patient in an intensive-care unit is provided with everything diagnostically necessary in an emergency—everything, that is, except the sense of security and ease that the body needs even more than pinpointed and clicking surveillance. It creates a tendency to panic, itself one of the most dangerous multipliers of disease. Many doctors are increasingly aware of the circular paradox of the intensive-care unit. It provides better electronic aids than ever before for dealing with emergencies that are often intensified because they communicate a sense of imminent disaster to the patient. It dramatizes the absence of warm contact between physician and patient.

Dr. Jerome D. Frank, of the Johns Hopkins University School of Medicine, told students at the university's graduating exercises in 1975 that any treatment of an illness that does not also minister to the human spirit is grossly deficient. He cited a 1974 British study showing that the survival rate of patients with heart disease being treated in an intensive-care unit was no higher than the survival rate of similar patients being treated at home. His interpretation was that the emotional strain of being surrounded by emergency electronic gadgets in an atmosphere of crisis offsets any theoretical technological gain.

In that same commencement talk, Dr. Frank referred to a study of 176 cases of cancer that remitted without surgery, X-rays, or chemotherapy. The question raised by these episodes was whether a powerful factor in those remissions may have been the deep belief by the patients that they were going to recover and their equally deep conviction that their doctors also believed they were going to recover.

One of the most succinct statements I have read anywhere bearing on the need of the patient to have faith in the physician was written by Dr. Robert R. Rynearson in the *Journal of Clinical Psychiatry*, June 1978. "Illness," wrote Dr. Rynearson, "particularly chronic illness, may force the sufferer into a dependent relationship with the person who offers to heal him. If trust does not become an important part of this relationship, it is unlikely that healing will occur. Physicians who ignore the importance of the relationship with the sufferer are often those who possess a simpleminded philosophy about illness—that is, that illness is the enemy which he assaults with all the skill and technology at his command. And, technology being what it is today, the sufferer may succumb to the treatment.

"Physicians need to be in actual touch with patients. Increasing technology in medicine is pushing the physician away from the patient. If the physician allows machinery to be interposed between him and the patient, he will be in danger of forfeiting powerful healing influences. A thorough physical examination fosters trust—there is a laying on of hands and a listening attitude. The sufferer is being touched and understood. The physician is then allowed to collaborate with the patient in altering the delicate balance between illness and health.

"Physicians must resist the idea that technology will some day abolish disease. As long as humans feel threatened and helpless, they will seek the sanctuary that illness provides. The distinguished scientist and humanitarian, Jacob Bronowski, cautioned us in this regard: 'We have to cure ourselves of the itch for absolute knowledge and power. We have to close the distance between the push-button order and the human act. We have to touch people.'"

Dr. Bernard Lown, professor of cardiology at the Harvard University School of Public Health, said in *Modern Medicine* magazine (September 30, 1978), that he believed it important for the physician to be present at the emergency room when his or her patient arrived. "Nothing is more decisive," he said, "in determining the outcome following a heart attack than for the patient to see his own physician. You can provide reassurance and psychological support at this crucial time in the patient's life.

"If you look at the total spectrum, 40 percent of

patients who have a heart attack die. And patients are aware of this fact and perceive they may be dying. . . . A second important principle is the laying on of hands—a practice that is rapidly atrophying because physicians are too busy with a laying on of tools. Both presence and touch help to establish a reassuring connection with the patient. I believe that physicians must recognize this profound truth before turning to drugs—the lidocaines, the morphines, the quinidines, and the like. So when I arrive, I say to the patient: 'Yes, you have had a heart attack, but you are going to recover.' And I'm very dogmatic about it even though the attack may be so massive that I have great trepidations about prognosis."

I musn't make it seem that medical technology does not represent a great boon in diagnosis and treatment. It is now possible, for example, to spare patients the ordeal of exploratory surgery because of a device that can enable the physician to peer directly into areas of the body that were not visible except by invasive procedures. The same device can be adapted to snip off harmful growths without having to perform deep surgery to get at them. Other machines are equally beneficial.

The problem with the new technology is that some practitioners tend to forget that these marvels can be intimidating to the patient, particularly when the last thing in the world the patient needs is another strange face or strange experience. Encounters with electronic gadgets call for careful psychological preparation, if the level of apprehension is not to be raised. All this requires time, of course. Time is the one thing that patients need most from their doctors—time to be heard, time to have things explained, time to be reassured, time to be introduced by the doctor personally to specialists or other attendants whose very existence seems to reflect something new and threatening. Yet the one thing that too many doctors find most difficult to command or manage is time. Indeed, some doctors tend to favor the new technology precisely because they don't have time enough to allow the diagnosis to emerge from comprehensive direct personal examination, and from extended give-and-take with the patient.

Sometimes a battery of tests will be given pro forma, even though the need for them is not clear. This can be expensive for the patient. Dr. Grey Dimond, provost of the school of medicine of the University of Missouri at Kansas City, sent me the copy of a bill for medical services received by an elderly woman of his acquaintance. I quote from Dr. Dimond's letter:

"The examining doctor had no compunction whatever in requesting $25.00 for an electrocardiogram; $20.00 for a ballistocardiogram (which is a useless procedure); $20.00 for an apexcardiogram (of no use in clinical practice); $35.00 for a vectocardiogram (totally of no recognized use in clinical medicine); $15.00 for a fluoroscopy (which he should not have been doing because of the risk to himself as well as the patient); $35.00 for a basal metabolism test (which is no longer done at teaching hospitals); and, finally, two urinalyses for $15.00 (I do not quarrel with these last two procedures simply because I do not know why they were ordered.)

"I send this bill along to you, realizing that one such doctor's billing proves nothing. I have watched this steadily happen, however, in American medicine, and you and I both know that the public is now highly vocal and greatly concerned over the disappearing attentiveness of the physician and the increasing mechanization of medical care. . . . When the physician placed himself on a fee schedule wherein he could justify his livelihood only by 'doing something,' he inevitably began shutting down the essence of a physician's purpose: the human contact.

"At the same time, he automatically placed himself at the disposal of a computer appraisal, and equally, permitted surgical procedures and mechanistic medicine to have premium positions on the fee-for-service scale. There has been no corresponding dollar return for the time spent in taking a detailed history and doing a slow and purposeful physical examination, and above all making the patient understand what has been done, why it was done, and what is the appropriate health care program."

The basic issue is not the usefulness of the new technology. It is the philosophical frame in which the new technology is brought into play and how it is used.

Perhaps the most serious consequence of the new technology is that it is pushing the doctor's little black bag out of style and, possibly, out of existence. Indeed, one of the reasons why so many doctors decline to make house calls is not just that out-of-office functions are too time-consuming, but that they no longer feel comfortable practicing out of a little black bag. They have allowed their skills to be harnessed to computers and exotic electronic diagnostic equipment.

Hundreds of letters from doctors about the *NEJM* article reflected the view that no medication they could give their patients was as potent as the state of mind that a patient brings to his or her own illness. In this sense, they said, the most valuable service a physician can provide to a patient is helping him to maximize his own recuperative and healing potentialities.

In my *NEJM* article I had allowed for the possibility that I might have been all wrong about the efficacy of ascorbic acid, and that I could have been the beneficiary of a self-administered placebo.

Dr. Bernard Ecanow and Dr. Bernard Gold, of the University of Illinois at the Medical Center, wrote to say that it was serious error for me to believe that the improvement in my condition after the systematic use of ascorbates was merely a placebo effect. They had done extensive research on the subject, and enclosed papers showing that ascorbate has a dispersal effect on clusters of red blood cells (RBCs). The reason my sedimentation rate had dropped after each intravenous dose of ascorbate, they said, was because it "produced dispersal of aggregated RBCs through its water structure breaking (hydophobic bond-breaking) effect, breaking up the structural water macromolecular matrix so that the RBCs are no longer held together by it."

I interpreted this explanation to mean that ascorbate was useful in restoring the chemical balances in the blood, or what Walter Cannon termed homeostasis.

Additional supporting data on the improvement in my condition after taking ascorbic acid came from the Lederle Research Laboratories. Drs. Arnold Oronsky and Suresh Kewar reported on research in their laboratories showing that ascorbic acid is essential for the proper functioning of prolylhydroxylase, which in turn is essential for the synthesis of collagen. The significance of ascorbate in the treatment of collagen diseases such as arthritis, therefore, seems compelling.

Earlier in this chapter, I referred to the work of Irwin Stone. With the exception of Albert Szent-Gyorgyi, Stone probably has probed more deeply into the phenomenon of ascorbic acid than any other medical researcher in the country.

Stone has attempted to account for the fact that the human species is unable to manufacture or store ascorbic acid, a vital ingredient in the immunological system installed by nature in all members of the animal kingdom except man and several other mammals.

Fascinated by this fact, Stone pursued his study of the subject both anthropologically and biochemically. He developed the theory that a genetic defect took place very early in the course of evolution: human beings lost their ability to make ascorbic acid and have had to depend on food containing the substance that plays so large a part in the immunological system. In areas where citrus fruits and certain vegetables were readily available, the regular diet compensated for the natural deficiency. In northern climes, however, the absence of citrus fruits resulted not just in scurvy but in increased susceptibility to a wide range of illnesses, minor and major.

Irwin Stone emphasizes that ascorbic acid, strictly speaking, is not a vitamin but a liver metabolite. Its primary reputation as a vitamin, however, has made it heir to the negative feelings of doctors because of the public's tendency to be attracted to miracle vitamin cures. Stone is hopeful that the medical profession will make a distinction between ascorbic acid and other vitamins not because he undervalues the need for adequate intake of vitamins but because the therapeutic properties of ascorbic acid play such a vital role in the healing process. With respect not just to poor diet but to an environment becoming increasingly burdened with air and water pollution, congestion, noise, and stress, the antitoxic role of ascorbic acid cannot be overestimated.

I must not make it appear that ascorbic acid can be taken indiscriminately and in limitless doses. Under certain circumstances, it can cause irritation to the digestive system. Such irritation, continued regularly over a long period, may be harmful and even dangerous. Ascorbic acid, especially in potent concentrations, should not be taken between meals. It is most effective when combined with bioflavinoids. It has a tendency to absorb vitamin B, therefore requires B complex supplementation. It also tends to chelate minerals out of the body. These characteristics can be highly valuable as a method of treating lead-poisoning or as an antidote to lead in the environment. But minerals other than lead are also chelated from the blood as the result of large doses of ascorbic acid.

One can understand the apprehensions of the medical profession about the notion that vitamins are the answer to any illness. Yet it is also true that some doctors have fostered the equally erroneous idea that the average supermarket shopping basket is insurance against any nutritional deficiency. Considering the preservatives, coloring agents, additives, and sugar overload in many processed foods, it is relevant to refer once again to the pronouncement of the White House Conference on Food, Nutrition, and Health, in 1969; namely, that one of the great failures in the education of medical students is the absence of adequate instruction in nutrition.

In any event, it was encouraging to me, in going through the mail from doctors, to see the growing evidence of a balanced attitude about nutrition in general and ascorbic acid in particular. The negative views held by many doctors only a few years ago are now being replaced by a willingness to examine new findings and to apply them in proper proportion.

It is also encouraging to know that the medical profession is giving increased emphasis to immunology and to the natural drive of the human body to heal itself. Considerable mystery still surrounds this process. As indicated in an earlier chapter, one of the interesting clues now being pursued is the function of ascorbic acid in serving both the immunological and healing processes. In this connection, it is worth calling attention to the current practice of many British hospitals of administering intravenous doses of ascorbic acid instead of antibiotics as a routine postoperative procedure in guarding against infection.

A number of doctors felt that my emphasis on the positive emotions was in accord with an important new trend in medicine. They said it was scientifically correct for me to state in the *NEJM* article that, just as the negative emotions produce negative chemical changes in the body, so the positive emotions are connected to positive chemical changes. My attention was called to papers by Dr. O. Carl Simonton on emotional stress as a cause of cancer, and by Dr. J. B. Imboden and Dr. A. Canter showing that moods of depression impair the body's immunological functions.

\* \* \*

A dozen or more telephone calls came from physicians who shared the article with patients whose will to live was not very robust. The physicians asked if I would telephone their patients and attempt to encourage them. This I tried to do to the best of my ability. One case in particular is perhaps worth mentioning. A physician told me about his patient, a young lady of twenty-three, who was gradually losing the use of her legs because of a collagen-related illness. She lived with her family in Atlanta. One of the psychological problems was that the entire family was becoming unhinged by worry and despair. Hospital care was out of the question because the insurance benefits had long since run out.

Her presence at home, her doctor told me, produced an atmosphere of apprehension and tension. The fact of her progressive paralysis was translated into the visible anguish of all concerned. It was essential, therefore, that some way be found to keep the entire family from disintegrating. The doctor believed that a positive change in the daughter's own feelings about herself was essential to any change for the better —not just in her own condition but in the collective health of the entire family. He had given her my article and she had responded so affirmatively that he felt a direct expression of interest from me would be useful. I telephoned the young lady, whom I shall call Carole. She spoke slowly but cogently as she described her difficulty, after two years, in believing that the paralysis would not become progressively worse until she would become totally disabled. Her doctor was trying to persuade her not to give up hope. He had told her that her medication and her exercises would work much better if she had goals in life and put her will to live fully to work.

I asked whether she thought this made good sense.

"It sounds fine in theory," she said, "but I don't think my doctor has ever been very ill himself, seriously ill, that is. He doesn't know how long a day can be, how difficult it is to have goals when nothing happens, how your mind turns on all the things that you aren't supposed to think about, like how you aren't getting any better and how week after week passes without any progress. You would understand it because you were there yourself. Weren't you terribly discouraged?"

I said I was, especially at the start when I expected my doctor to fix my body as though it were an automobile engine that needed mechanical repair, like cleaning out the carburetor, or reconnecting the fuel pump. But then I realized that a human being is not a machine—and only a human being has a built-in mechanism for repairing itself, for ministering to its own needs, and for comprehending what is happening to it. The regenerative and restorative force in human beings is at the core of human uniqueness. Sometimes this force is blocked or underdeveloped. One of the most important things a doctor can do for a patient is to assess the capacity of each individual to put that force fully to work. Carole's doctor was giving her important advice when he told her that his treatment would work best when combined with the natural drive of the body to right itself.

I was also fortunate, I said, in having a doctor who believed that my own will to live would actually set the stage for progress; he encouraged me in everything I did for myself.

Carole said she was curious about the laughter. Was it really as important in my recovery as the article had indicated?

What was significant about the laughter, I said, was not just the fact that it provides internal exercise for

145

ANATOMY OF AN ILLNESS

a person flat on his or her back—a form of jogging for the innards—but that it creates a mood in which the other positive emotions can be put to work, too. In short, it helps make it possible for good things to happen.

Carole wanted to know how she could find things worth laughing about. I said she would have to work at it, just as she would have to work at anything else worthwhile. I suggested that members of the family ought to take turns going to the library, for example, in order to find books with genuine laugh-producing qualities. I wasn't thinking just of joke books by collectors such as Bennett Cerf—although I doubt that I have ever known anyone who was more systematic about pursuing good stories than Bennett, who once contributed a regular column on publishing to SR— a column that always managed to include a story or two worth retelling. I told Carole that I had in mind writers like Stephen Leacock and Ogden Nash and James Thurber and Ludwig Bemelmans. I also suggested books like Max Eastman's *Enjoyment of Laughter,* and the Whites' *Subtreasury of American Humor.* In any case, I was certain she and other members of the family would enjoy tracking down these and other books, and I hoped she would look into the humor of other cultures.

Carole brightened at these suggestions. Then I told her she could do something for me. She could pick out one of these stories each day and share it with me. Specifically, I suggested that she telephone me at 9:30 A.M. every day and tell me what she and the family regarded as the best of the day's crop.

Then I spoke to Carole's mother, who fell in with the idea. She said she would develop a plan under which each of the members of the family would take turns going to the library or the book store, for material the entire family could examine. Everyone would then join in the voting for the story to be read to me over the telephone by Carole.

Two days later, the plan was in full operation. Carole telephoned. Her voice was vibrant. She was laughing even before she could finish her first sentence.

"I don't know whether I'm going to be able to get this out," she said. "Even before calling you I tried to rehearse so I wouldn't laugh before I reached the punch line, and I broke up each time. I'll probably wet the bed before I get through. We did some research on the kinds of stories that might interest you. You play golf, don't you? At least I read somewhere that you occasionally play with Arnold Palmer and that you perpetuated some spoofs on golf in *Saturday Review*."

I confessed to an inept acquaintance with the sport.

"Well, there was this priest who was playing golf," she said, "and he had difficulty in hitting the ball over a small pond. After he put five balls in the water, he hesitated before teeing up again, then said to his caddy: 'I know what I'm doing wrong. I just forgot to pray before each shot, that was all.' He prayed, then swung at the ball—and it traveled about twenty yards in a loop right into the water. 'Father,' asked the caddy, 'might I make a suggestion?' 'Certainly, son,' the priest said. 'Well, father,' the caddy said, 'the next time you pray, keep your head down.' "

It was one of the oldest stories in the history of golf, but it was new to Carole and I joined in her unrestrained laughter. Then she told me that most of the fun came during the family discussion the previous afternoon, when they considered a dozen or more stories before deciding on the one she would tell. "It was wonderful," Carole said. "My mother came back from the library with about a dozen books and she had the time of her life acting out some of the funny stories. She always wanted to go on the stage anyway. Well, after she completed her act, we all voted for our favorite. My brother took his turn in the library this morning. He's more literary than the rest of us. He'll probably come back with passages from O. Henry or Mark Twain or a short story, so get ready for a long session the next time I call."

What pleased me most about the incident was that the family was finding a new and far more pleasant connection to Carole. The fact that they had been able to be collectively engaged in a joyous enterprise involving Carole was as important to them as it was to her. When Carole's doctor telephoned two days later, it was this new aspect of the family situation that pleased him most. He said that his visit to the home almost startled him, for the faces were no longer morose and furrowed but open and expectant. Members of the family competed with one another in telling him what they were doing and even made him vote on the next story that Carole should tell me.

Two weeks later, the doctor telephoned again to say he felt the big gain that had been scored was in the quality of life for the entire family. It was too early to say anything about Carole's physical condition, but it seemed clear to him that she had much more energy and was definitely more hopeful.

The central point the doctor had made about the quality of life is worth stressing. Not every illness can be overcome. But many people allow illness to disfigure their lives more than it should. They cave in needlessly. They ignore and weaken whatever powers they may have for standing erect. There is always a margin within which life can be lived with meaning and even with a certain measure of joy, despite illness. Not all serious and even fatal illnesses are accompanied by high fever and unremitting pain. It is possible, therefore, for at least as much emphasis to be placed on the quality of life as on treatment.

This principle was underlined for me by a New York City doctor who telephoned to say he had terminal cancer. He said he had been prompted by the *NEJM* article to try to get the most out of life while he was still mobile and capable of making direct contact with all the things that gave him pleasure.

"I don't think I would dare suggest to others what I am doing for myself," he said. "There is such a strong tradition to do battle against cancer with all the technology and chemotherapy at our command that we seldom have the time or the courage to ask other important questions—questions involving values. Are

149

we justified, for example, in going at a terminal cancer victim with chemotherapy and radiation that will produce all sorts of enfeebling complications, just because of the possibility that we might be better able, hypothetically, to add a few months to a patient's life? Or is it better for that individual to use every minute of that time in ways that are rewarding and life-giving? The choice was easy for me. I am now doing many of the things I always wanted to do. I can't be too strenuous, of course, but it is surprising how active I can be compared to the immobility I had feared.

"What I do for myself comes out of my philosophy, not out of my science. Once I depart from science in the treatment of others, I am in another field entirely —one for which ministers and psychologists are perhaps better qualified than I. It is something of a dilemma for me, but I am attempting, even within the context of traditional treatment, to upgrade the spirits of my patients. I've had a great deal of luck in getting them to take humor seriously"—he chuckled over his juxtaposition—"and I thought you might be interested in knowing that it works very well. I don't hesitate to tell them that I've got the same problem as they do. When they see me laugh, they almost feel ashamed of themselves if they are incapable of doing the same. My sessions with my patients are anything but grim. I want them to look forward to my coming. I want to look forward to being with them. And I just wanted you to know that what you said about laughter in the *NEJM* is just fine with me."

What was most striking about his account was that

his perception of his duty as a medical scientist was in conflict with his philosophical convictions on the art of living. He felt bound by his training to confine himself to the treatment of disease. Yet his own problem and the problem of his patients transcended disease at a certain point and involved basic values in living. His solution to his own problem was to put the quality of life ahead of the kind of scientific treatment that was generally prescribed in cases such as his own.

Many writers throughout history have had different interpretations of this general dilemma, Tolstoy, Dostoyevsky, Molière, and G.B. Shaw among them. Is life to be prolonged under conditions of extreme suffering? Does the doctor have the obligation to fight disease with every weapon at his disposal, even though the weapons he uses will levy a heavy tax on the way a person feels?

Other dilemmas have to do with the need to decide which life to save where the doctor can save only one, such as the case of mother and child. The dilemma of the doctor to whom I had spoken was perhaps the most vexing of all. How far does he go beyond his own discipline in applying what he himself believes to be true? Is there a conflict at times between the treatment of disease and the treatment of human beings?

Many medical schools are now dealing with questions such as these. The decade of the 1970s has seen an important new awareness of the need to prepare medical students not just for the profession of medical science but for dealing with abstract issues continually being created by new knowledge and by a fast-developing technology. The National Endowment for the Humanities, created by an act of Congress, has appropriated many millions of dollars for the development of courses on medical ethics. At least fifty schools of medicine have benefitted from NEH grants in this area. The Hastings Foundation has undertaken perhaps the most comprehensive studies in the field of medical ethics of any private organization. A number of leaders in medical education have formed an organization, the Society for Health and Human Values, which serves as a center not just for the development of ethics and values in the curriculum of medical schools, but as an exchange post for those inside and outside the medical profession. Another important development in this field is the establishment at Columbia University's College of Physicians and Surgeons of *Man & Medicine,* a quarterly journal of ethics and values.

* * *

Earlier in this chapter, I wrote about Carole's apprehension that her doctor might not understand what it was like to be seriously ill and on a downslope. The idea is worth pursuing.

In his book, *Out of My Life and Thought,* Albert Schweitzer wrote about his own serious illness in early middle age, and his conviction at the time that if he ever recovered he would never forget his own feelings while ill; he would try as a doctor to give at least as much attention to the psychology of the patient as he did to a diagnosis. There is a "fellowship of those who bear the mark of pain," Schweitzer wrote in his book. Those outside this fellowship have great difficulty in comprehending what lies behind the pain.

I know that, during my own illness in 1964, my fellow patients at the hospital would talk about matters they would never discuss with their doctors. The psychology of the seriously ill put barriers between us and those who had the skill and the grace to minister to us.

There was first of all the feeling of helplessness— a serious disease in itself.

There was the subconscious fear of never being able to function normally again—and it produced a wall of separation between us and the world of open movement, open sounds, open expectations.

There was the reluctance to be thought a complainer.

There was the desire not to add to the already great burden of apprehension felt by one's family; this added to the isolation.

There was the conflict between the terror of loneliness and the desire to be left alone.

There was the lack of self-esteem, the subconscious feeling perhaps that our illness was a manifestation of our inadequacy.

There was the fear that decisions were being made behind our backs, that not everything was made known that we wanted to know, yet dreaded knowing.

There was the morbid fear of intrusive technology, fear of being metabolized by a data base, never to regain our faces again. There was resentment of strangers who came at us with needles and vials—some of which put supposedly magic substances in our veins, and others which took more of our blood than we thought we could afford to lose. There was the distress of being wheeled through white corridors to laboratories for all sorts of strange encounters with compact machines and blinking lights and whirling discs.

And there was the utter void created by the longing—ineradicable, unremitting, pervasive—for warmth of human contact. A warm smile and an outstretched hand were valued even above the offerings of modern science, but the latter were far more accessible than the former.

I became convinced that nothing a hospital could provide in the way of technological marvels was as helpful as an atmosphere of compassion. Also, continuity of personnel. Well-to-do patients are generally in a position to protect themselves against a long procession of different faces; they can hire medical attendants according to any standards they may wish to apply. But for most people the facts of hospital life involve discontinuity, fractioned care, and inadequate protection against surprise. People come and go; you make your adjustments as best you can.

The central question to be asked about hospitals— or about doctors for that matter—is whether they inspire the patient with the confidence that he or she is in the right place; whether they enable him to have trust in those who seek to heal him; in short, whether he has the expectation that good things will happen.

\* \* \*

Several doctors wrote to ask whether I had been influenced in my decision to use large doses of ascorbic acid by the statements and writings of Linus Pauling. My experience with ascorbic acid occurred in 1964. Dr. Pauling's first major work on ascorbic acid *(Vitamin C and the Common Cold)* appeared in 1970. After the publication of that work, I wrote to Linus Pauling about the episode. Since that time, we have corresponded and I have followed his research in this field with great interest.

Some of the letters from doctors asked whether there had been anything in my medical history to prepare me psychologically and philosophically for the "partnership" with Dr. Hitzig in the diagnosis and treatment of my illness in 1964. There were two such episodes.

My first experience in coping with a bleak medical diagnosis came at the age of ten, when I was sent to a tuberculosis sanitarium. I was terribly frail and underweight, and it seemed logical to suppose that I was in the grip of a serious malady. Later it was discovered that the doctors had mistakenly interpreted normal calcification as TB markings. X-rays at that time were not yet a totally reliable basis for complex diagnosis. In any case, I spent six months at the sanitarium.

What was most interesting to me about that early experience was that patients divided themselves into two groups: those who were confident they would beat back the disease and be able to resume normal lives, and those who resigned themselves to a prolonged and even fatal illness. Those of us who held to the optimistic view became good friends, involved ourselves in creative activities, and had little to do with the patients who had resigned themselves to the worst. When newcomers arrived at the hospital, we did our best to recruit them before the bleak brigade went to work.

I couldn't help being impressed with the fact that the boys in my group had a far higher percentage of "discharged as cured" outcomes than the kids in the other group. Even at the age of ten, I was being philosophically conditioned; I became aware of the power of the mind in overcoming disease. The lessons I learned about hope at that time played an important part in my complete recovery and in the feelings I have had since about the preciousness of life.

By the time I was seventeen, I had completely overcome the early frailty. I had fallen in love with vigorous sports; year by year my body continued to grow and harden. This addiction to sports stayed with me. I have also had the advantage of being married to a woman who is endowed with a blessed cheerfulness and who believes deeply in the advantages of good nutrition.

The second major episode occurred during 1954, in my thirty-ninth year. With increased family responsibilities, I thought it prudent to apply for additional insurance. The company doctors turned me down, saying the cardiograms showed evidence of a serious coronary occlusion. My aunt, who was the insurance agent, was completely frank about the findings of the doctors. Despite the absence of active supporting evidence, they diagnosed an "ischemic" condition, characterized by a thickening of the walls of the heart and an erratic heartbeat. She said they urgently advised me to give up almost everything and to take to my bed for several months. I felt demolished by this report. It was inconceivable that I would have to give up my job, my travels, and an active sports life. But here was my aunt telling me that the insurance doctors said that if I became completely inactive, I might be able to stretch out my life for a year and a half.

I decided to say nothing to my wife about the verdict of the insurance doctors. When I came home that night, my little daughters came running up to me. They liked to be thrown high in the air and to dive from my shoulders onto the couch. For a split second, I looked down two roads. One was marked "cardiac alley." If I accepted the advice of the specialists, I would never throw my girls in the air again. The second road would find me working full tilt at *SR* and doing all the other things that spelled life to me. The second road might carry me for a few months or a few weeks or a few minutes; but it was my road. It was an easy decision. I caught my little girls as they came running up to me and threw them higher in the air than ever before. The next day I played in a singles tennis tournament for perhaps a total of forty-five or fifty games.

The following Monday I telephoned Dr. Hitzig

157

and informed him of the grim verdict of the insurance doctors. He ordered me to his office immediately, then took me to the chief of cardiology at Mount Sinai Hospital. The hospital cardiograms confirmed the insurance reports. I went back to Bill Hitzig's office. We had a good talk. I told him I intended to do exactly what I had been doing all along and that I doubted there was any cardiograph in the world that knew everything that had to be known about what made my heart tick. Hitzig patted me on the back and said he was behind me all the way.

Three years later I met Paul Dudley White, the famed heart specialist. He listened carefully to the account of what had happened, then told me that I had done the only thing that could have saved my life. He believed that sustained and vigorous exercise was necessary for the proper functioning of the human heart, even when there was evidence of the kind of cardiac inefficiency that had been diagnosed in my case. He said that if I had accepted the verdict of the specialists in 1954, I probably would have confirmed it.

That meeting with Paul Dudley White was something of a landmark in my life. It gave me confidence in my rapport with my own body. It reinforced my conviction that the human mind can discipline the body, can set goals for itself, can somehow comprehend its own potentiality and move resolutely forward.

In recounting this episode, I certainly do not intend to suggest that patients with serious heart disease should go against the advice of their doctors. I had Dr.

Hitzig's backing. Besides, there were factors in my case that might not apply to others.

Has my respect for the medical profession diminished as the result of the three episodes? Just the opposite. The thousands of letters I have received from doctors have demolished any notion that physicians are universally resistant to psychological, moral, or spiritual factors in the healing process. Most doctors recognize that medicine is just as much an art as it is a science and that the most important knowledge in medicine to be learned or taught is the way the human mind and body can summon innermost resources to meet extraordinary challenges.

Some of the letters asked whether I would be able, in the event of another serious illness, to mount the kind of total response that I did earlier in my life.

My answer was that I honestly don't know how many such efforts are possible in a single lifetime. But I know I would certainly try.

I know I have been lucky. My body has already carried me far beyond the point where the medical experts in 1954 thought it would go. According to my calculations, my heart has furnished me with 876,-946,280 more heartbeats than were thought possible by the insurance doctors.

It was the sheerest of coincidences that, on the tenth anniversary of my 1964 illness, I should happen to meet on the street in New York one of the specialists who had made the melancholy diagnosis of progressive paralysis. He was clearly surprised to see me. I held out my hand. He took it. I didn't hold back on the handshake. I had a point I wanted to make, and I thought the best way to do so was through a greeting firm enough to make an impression. I increased the pressure until he winced and asked to be released. He said he could tell from my handshake that he didn't have to ask about my present condition, but he was eager to hear what was behind the recovery.

It all began, I said, when I decided that some experts don't really know enough to make a pronouncement of doom on a human being. And I said I hoped they would be careful about what they said to others; they might be believed and that could be the beginning of the end.

# BIBLIOGRAPHY

*Acupuncture anesthesia.* Translation of a Chinese publication of the same title. Bethesda, Maryland: National Institutes of Health, 1975.

Adler, H. The doctor-patient relationship revisited. *Ann. Internal Med.* 78:4, April 1973, p. 595.

Akil, H., et al. Enkephalin like material elevated in ventricular cerebrospinal fluid of pain patients after analgetic focal stimulation. *Science* 201 (4354): 463–65, August 4, 1978.

Aletky, et al. Sex differences and placebo effects: motivation as an intervening variable. *J. Consulting and Clinical Psych.* 43:2, 1975.

Alexander, F. *Psychosomatic medicine.* New York: W. W. Norton and Company, 1950.

Alvarez, W.C. *Minds that came back.* New York: J.B. Lippincott, 1961.

Basolwitz, H.; Persky, H.; Korchin, S.J.; and Grinkler, R.R. *Anxiety and stress.* New York: McGraw-Hill, 1955.

Beckman, B.L. Life stress and psychological well being. *J. Health and Social Behavior* 12: 35–45, 1971.

Beecher, H.K. Evidence for increased effectiveness of placebos with increased stress. *Am. J. Physiology* 187:163(b), 1956.

———. The powerful placebo. *JAMA* 159: 1602–06, 1955.

Bell, B.D. Cognitive dissonance and life satisfaction of older adults. *J. Gerontology* 29(5), 564–71, 1974.

Benson, Herbert, et al. The placebo effect: a neglected asset in the care of patients. *JAMA* 232:12, June 23, 1975.

Birk, L., ed. *Biofeedback: behavioral medicine.* New York: Grune and Stratton, 1973.

Birren, J.E., et al. Human aging: a biological and behavioral study. DHEW Publication No. (HSM) 71–9051, 1974.

Blackwell, B., et al. Demonstration to medical students of placebo responses and non drug factors. *Lancet,* June 1972, p. 1279.

163

# BIBLIOGRAPHY

Blake, K. Vitamin C: the case looks stronger, but. . . . *Pastimes* (shuttle edition). Eastern Airlines: March 1976.

Bloom, S.W., et al. Physician-patient expectations in primary care. *Bull. N.Y. Acad. Med.* 53(1) 75–82, January-February 1977.

Blum, R. *The management of the doctor-patient relationship.* New York: McGraw-Hill, 1960.

Bogdonoff, M.D., et al. The doctor-patient relationship. *JAMA* 192:1, April 5, 1965, p. 131.

Bok, S. The ethics of giving placebos. *Scientific American* 231:5, November 1974, p. 17.

Bond, M.R. Psychological and psychiatric aspects of pain. *Anaesthesia* 33(4): 355–61, April 1978.

Bonica, J.J. *The management of pain.* Philadelphia: Lea & Febiger, 1953.

Bonica, J.J., et al. *Advances in pain research and therapy*, vol. I. New York: Ravens Press, 1976.

Brand, P. Rehabilitation in leprosy (videotape recording). Washington: produced for the Bureau of Medical Services, Division of Hospitals, 1961.

Bromberg, W. An analysis of therapeutic artfulness. *Am. J. Psychiatry* 114, 1958, p. 719.

Brown, B. *New mind, new body.* New York: Harper and Row, 1975.
————. *Stress and the art of biofeedback.* New York: Harper and Row, 1977.

Burch, G.E. Of bellyache. *Am. Heart J.* 94(5): 668, November 1977.

Burton, R. *The anatomy of melancholy* (1621). Edited by Floyd Dell and Paul Jordan-Smith. New York: Tudor Publishing Company, 1941.

Cabot, R.C., and Dicks, R.L. *The art of ministering to the sick.* New York: Macmillan, 1936.

Cameron, E. Biological function of ascorbic acid and the pathogenesis of scurvy: a working hypothesis. *Med. Hypotheses* 3: 154–63, 1976.
————. *Hyaluronidase and cancer.* Oxford and New York: Pergamon Press, 1966.
————. Vitamin C. *Brit. I. Hosp. Med.* 13: 511, 1976.

Cameron, E., and Baird, G. Ascorbic acid and dependence on opiates in patients with advanced disseminated cancer. *J. Intern. Res. Commun.* I (96): 38, 1973.

Cameron, E., and Campbell, A. The orthomolecular treatment of cancer: II. Clinical trial of high-dose ascorbic acid supplements in advanced human cancer. *Chem.-Biol. Interact.* 9: 285–315, 1974.

Cameron, E.; Campbell, A.; and Jack, T. The orthomolecular

treatment of cancer: III. Reticulum cell sarcoma: double complete regression induced by high-dose ascorbic acid therapy. *Chem.-Biol. Interact.* III: 387–93, 1975.

Cameron, E., and Pauling, L. Ascorbic acid and the glycosaminoglycans; an orthomolecular approach to cancer and other diseases. *Oncology* 27: 181–92, 1973.

———. Supplemental ascorbate in the supportive cancer. *Proceedings of the National Academy of Sciences USA* 73: 3685–89, 1976.

Cameron, E., and Rotman, D. Ascorbic acid, cell proliferation, and cancer. *Lancet* I: 542, 1972.

Campbell, A. Subjective measures of well-being. *American Psychologist,* 117–24, 1976.

Cannon, W.B. *The wisdom of the body.* New York: W.W. Norton and Company, 1963.

Carter, A.B. The placebo, its use and abuse. *Lancet,* October 17, 1973, p. 823.

Castiglioni, A. *A history of medicine.* Translated from the Italian and edited by E.B. Krumbhaar. 2d ed., rev. and enl. New York: Knopf, 1947.

Cochrane, A.L. Effectiveness and efficiency: random reflections on health services. Nuffield Provincial Hospital Trust, 1974.

Comaroff, J. A bitter pill to swallow; placebo therapy in general practice. *Sociological Review* 24(1):79, February 1976.

Corson, S.A. Psychological stress and target tissue. In *Psychological aspects of cancer,* ed. E.M. Weyer and H. Hutchins. New York: New York Academy of Sciences, 1966, pp. 890–915.

Curro, F.A. The peripheral nervous system and its role in mediating pain. *Dent. Clin. North Am.* 22(1): 51–61, January 1978.

Cushing, H. *The life of Sir William Osler,* 2 vols. New York: Oxford University Press, 1940.

Danner, S., and Dunning, A. Spared affluence, they've lived past 90. *Medical World News,* January 23, 1978, 42.

De Sousa, C., et al. Pain: a review and interpretation. *Inst. J. Neurosci.* 7(2): 81–101, 1977.

Dlin, B.M. Risk factors, life style, and the emotions in coronary disease. *Psychosomatics,* October 1977, 28–31.

Dodge, D.L., and Martin, W.T. *Social stress and illness.* Notre Dame, Indiana: University of Notre Dame Press, 1970.

Dubner, R. Neurophysiology of pain. *Dent. Clin. North Am.* 22(1): 11–30, January 1978.

Dubos, R. *Man adapting.* New Haven: Yale University Press, 1965.

———. *Man, medicine and environment.* New York: Praeger, 1968.

———. Medicine's living history. *Medical World News,* 77–85, 1975.

————. *Mirage of health.* New York: Harper and Row, 1971.

————. The state of health and the quality of life. *Western J. of Medicine* 125(1), 8–9, July 1976.

Dubos, R.; Pines, M.; and Editors of *Life. Health and disease.* New York: Time/Life, 1965.

Dunbar, F. *Emotions and bodily changes.* New York: Columbia University Press, 1954.

Eastman, M. *The enjoyment of laughter.* Johnson reprint of 1937 edition. New York: Johnson Reprint Company, 1971.

Ecanow, B., and Gold, B.H. Erythrocyte sedimentation rates and malignancy: role of age and erythrocyte aggregation. *Science* 193, September 3, 1976, pp. 919–20.

Everson, T.C., and Cole, H. *Spontaneous regression of cancer.* Philadelphia: W. B. Saunders, 1966.

Ewin, D.M. Relieving suffering and pain with hypnosis. *Geriatrics* 33(6): 87–89, June 1978.

Fabrega, H., Jr., et al. Culture, language and the shaping of illness: an illustration based on pain. *J. Psychosom. Res.* 20(4): 323–37, 1976.

"Family doctor." Demand for, and definition of, "family doctor" (letter). *NEJM* 275(20): 1144–46, November 11, 1976.

Fligor, L. The placebo effect. (Letter in response to *JAMA* commentary.) *JAMA* 234:8 November 24, 1975.

Frank, J. The faith that heals. *Johns Hopkins Med. J.* 137: 127–31, 1975.

Freud, S. *Complete psychological works.* Translated from the German under the general editorship of James Strachey, in collaboration with Anna Freud, assisted by Alix Strachey and Alan Tyson. New York: W.W. Norton and Company, 1976.

Fry, W.F., Jr. The respiratory components of mirthful laughter. *J. Biol. Psychology* 19:2, 39–50, 1977.

Gardner, K., and Montgomery, P.S. *Clinical biofeedback: a procedural manual.* Baltimore: Williams and Wilkins, 1977.

Gold, H. *Cornell conferences on therapy,* vol. 1. Edited by H. Gold with others. New York: Macmillan, 1946.

Goodfield, J. Humanity in Science: a perspective and a plea. *Science* 198, 580–85, 1977.

Green, E. *Beyond biofeedback.* New York: Delacorte, 1977.

Green, J. On how to live 90 to 100 healthy years (the syndrome of longevity . . . its 7 great constants). *Executive Health* 6(10), 1974.

Greenberg, J. The stress-illness link: not "if" but "how." *Science News* 112: 394–98, 1977.

Greenleigh, L. Timelessness and restitution in relation to creativity and the aging process. *J. Am. Geriatrics Soc.* 8: 353, 1960.

Gunderson, E.K., and Rahe, R.H., eds. *Life stress and illness.* Springfield, Illinois: Charles C. Thomas, 1974.

Hamburger, E. A two-stage study of plasma ascorbic acid and its relation to wound healing. *Milit. Med.* 127: 723–25, 1962.

Handfield-Jones. A bottle of medicine from the doctor. *Lancet,* October 17, 1973, p. 823.

Hankoff, et al. Placebo response in schizophrenic outpatients *Arch. of Gen. Psychiatry* 2, January 1960, pp. 33, 43.

Hannay, D.R., et al. The use and perception of a health centre. *Practitioner* 218 (1304): 260–66, February 1977.

Harkins, W.W. Age and sex differences in pain perception. In *Pain in trigeminal region,* ed. D. J. Anderson and B. Matthews. New York: Elsevier-North Holland, 1977, pp. 435–41.

Henderson, L. J. Introductory lecture to sociology 23. Harvard University, c. 1930.

Hirsh, J.; Street, D.; and Cade, J.F., et al. Relation between bleeding time and platelet connective tissue reaction after aspirin. *Blood* 41: 369–77, March 1973.

Holden, C. Pain control with hypnosis. *Science* 198 (4319): 808, November 25, 1977.

Hospital stress and patient reports of pain and physical status. *J. Human Stress* 4(2): 28–37, June 1978.

Imboden, J.B.; Canter, A.; and Cluff, L.E. Convalescence from influenza. *Arch. Internal Med.* 103: 393, 1961.

Ingelfinger, F.J. Those anti-doctor books (letter to editor). *NEJM* February 1976, pp. 442–43.

James, W. *Psychology.* New York: World Publishing Company, 1948.

Jong, R.H. Central pain mechanisms. *JAMA* 239(26): 2784, June 30, 1978.

Keele, K.D. *Anatomies of pain.* Springfield, Illinois: Charles C. Thomas, 1957.

Kellgrin, J.H. Pain in the rheumatic diseases. *Rep. Rheum. Dis.* (61): 1–2, July 1977.

Kerwar, S.S. and Felix, A.M. The effect of L-34-dehydroproline on collagen synthesis and prolyl-hydroxylase activity in mammalian cell cultures. *J. Biolog. Chem.* 251: 503, 1976.

Kinderlehrer, J. Vitamin C: the best thing that ever happened to antibiotics. *Prevention* 26: 71–75, 1974.

Klenner, F.R. Observations on the dose and administration of ascorbic acid when employed beyond the range of a vitamin in human pathology. *J. Appl. Nutr.* 23: 61–87, 1971.

Krantz, J.C., Jr. The rendezvous with pain and home remedies, with special reference to the origins of aspirin. *J. Am. Med. Wom. Assoc.* 33(5): 223–24, May 1978.

*Lancet* editorial. The humble humbug. August 14, 1951, p. 321.

Landau, E., et al. Creativity and self-actualization in the aging personality. *Am. J. Psychother.* 32(1): 117–27, January 1978.

Lasagna, L. Placebos. *Scientific American* 193:68, 1956.

Lehman, H.C. *Age and achievement.* Princeton: Princeton University Press, 1953.

Levi, L. *Society, stress and disease.* New York: Oxford University Press, 1971.

Levine, C.I.; Aleo, J.; Prynne, C.; and Bates, C. Activation of proto-collagen proline-hydroxylase by ascorbic acid and cultured 3T6 fibroblasts. *Biochemica et Biophysica Acta* 29.

Levine, J.D.; Gordon, N.C.; and Fields, H.L. The mechanism of placebo analgesia. *Lancet* September 23, 1978, pp. 654–57.

Lipowski, Z.J. Psychosomatic medicine in the seventies: an overview. *Am. J. Psychiatry* 134(3), 1977.

Lown, B., and Segal, J. Post-MI care: how to manage your patient's arrhythmias. *Modern Medicine* 46:16, pp. 60–77.

Luce, G.G. *Body time.* New York: Bantam, 1973.

Luthe, W. *Creativity mobilization techniques.* New York: Grune and Stratton, 1976.

Maltbie, A.A., et al. A diagnostic approach to pain. *Psychosomatics* 19(6): 359–66, June 1978.

Melzack, R. *The puzzle of pain.* New York: Basic Books, Inc., 1973.

Melzack, R., and Wall, P.D. Pain mechanisms, a new theory. *Science* 150: 971–79, 1965.

Menninger, K., with M. Mayman and P. Pruyser. *The vital balance: the life process in mental health and illness.* New York: The Viking Press, 1963.

Menninger, R.W. Psychiatry 1976: time for a holistic medicine. *Ann. of Intern. Med.* 84(5), 603–04, May 1976.

Miller, J.Z., et al. Therapeutic effect of vitamin C. *JAMA* 237(3): 248–51, 1977.

Moody, R. A., Jr. *Laugh after laugh.* Jacksonville, Florida: Headwaters Press, 1978.

Morris, L., et al. Drug-name familiarity and the placebo effect. *J. Clinical Psych.* 30, July 1974, pp. 280–82.

Newell, K.W., ed. *Health by the people.* Geneva: World Health Organization, 1975.

Novosti Press Agency. Very old people in the USSR. *Gerontologist* 10(2), 151–52, 1970.

Older, J. Pain and the physician. *Post. Grad. Med.* 62(5): 3539, November 1977.

On opiates, pain and the nervous system (editorial). *Neurosurgery* 1(2): 188–89, September-October 1977.

Osler, W. *Aequanimitas.* New York: McGraw-Hill, 1906.

Owen, A. *Hysteria, hypnosis and healing: the work of J.M.Charcot.* New York: Garrett Publications-Helix Press, 1970.

Pace, J.B. Psychophysiology of pain: diagnostic and therapeutic implications. *J. Fam. Pract.* 5(4): 553–57, October 1977.

Pain: selected bibliography. *Pain* 4(4), April 1978, pp. 379–91.

Pain sensation in man (editorial). *Brit. Med. J.* 2(6090): 783–84, September 24, 1977.

Park, C.C., and Shapiro, L.N. You are not alone. Boston and Toronto: Little, Brown and Company, 1976.

Paskind, H.A. Effect of laughter on muscle tone. *Arch. Neurol. and Psychiatry* 28: 623–28, 1932.

Pauling, L. *Vitamin C and the common cold.* San Francisco: W.H. Freeman, 1970.

Peace at the last (editorial). *Lancet* 1(8066): 698–700, April 1, 1978.

Pelletier, K.R. *Holistic medicine.* New York: Delacorte, forthcoming.

————. *Mind as healer, mind as slayer:* a holistic approach to preventing stress disorders. New York: Delacorte, 1977.

————. *Toward a science of consciousness.* New York: Delacorte, 1978.

Penfield, W. *The mystery of the mind.* Princeton: Princeton University Press, 1975.

Perl, E.R. Is pain a specific sensation? *J. Psychiatri. Res.* 8: 273–87, 1971.

Petersdorf, R.G. The doctor's dilemma *NEJM* 299 (12) 628–34, September 21, 1978.

Picaza, J.A., et al. Pain suppression: chronic effects. *Neurosurgery* 1(2): 226–27, September-October 1977.

Pilowsky, I. Pain as abnormal illness behavior. *J. Human Stress* 4(2): 22–27, June 1978.

Pilowsky, I., et al. Pain, depression and illness behavior in a pain clinic population. *Pain* 4(2): 183–92, December 1977.

Popenoe, C. *Wellness.* New York: Random House, 1977.

Poznamski, E.O. Children's reactions to pain: a psychiatrist's perspective. *Clin. Pediatr.* 15(12): 114–19, December 1976.

Relman, A.S. Holistic medicine (editorial). *NEJM* 300:6, 1979, pp. 312–13.

————. Who will train all those primary care physicians (editorial). *NEJM* 299(12): 652–53, September 21, 1978.

Roueché, B. Annals of medicine: placebo. *New Yorker*, October 15, 1960.

Rynearson, R.R. Touching people (editorial). *J. Clin. Psychiatry* 39(6): 492, June 1978.

Sahud, M.A., and Cohen, R.J. Effect of aspirin ingestion on ascorbic-acid levels in rheumatoid arthritis. *Lancet* 1: 937–38, 1971.

Schweitzer, A. *Out of my life and thought, an autobiography.* Translated by C. T. Campion. New York: Holt, 1949.

Selye, H. *From dream to discovery.* Montreal, Canada: International Institute of Stress, 1975.

————. *The stress of life.* New York: McGraw-Hill, 1956.

Shapiro, A.K. Factors contributing to the placebo effect. *Am. J. Psychother.* 18, 1961, pp. 73–88.

————. The placebo effect in the history of medical treatment: implications for psychiatry. *Am. J. Psychiatry* 116: 298, 1959.

Silverman, S. *Psychologic cues in forecasting physical illness.* New York: Appleton Century, 1970.

Simon, R.K. Freud's concepts of comedy and suffering. *Psychoanal. Rev.* 64(3): 391–407, Fall 1977.

Simonton, D.K. Creative productivity, age and stress: a biographical time-series analysis of 10 classical composers. *J. Pers. Soc. Psychol.* 35(11): 791–804, November 1977.

Simonton, O.C., and Matthews-Simonton, S. Belief systems and management of the emotional aspects of malignancy. *J. Transpersonal Psychology* 7(1), 29–47, 1975.

Single, G. Pathway for pain—some anatomical and clinical considerations. *Med. J. Malaysia* 32(2): 152–56, December 1977.

Smith, A. *Powers of the mind.* New York: Random House, 1975, pp. 11–14.

Sperryn, P.N.; Hamilton, E.B.; and Parsons, V. Double-blind comparison of aspirin and 4-(acetamido) phenyl-2-acetoxy-benzoate (benorylate) in rheumatoid arthritis. *Ann. Rheum. Dis.* 32: 157–61, March 1973.

Sternbach, R.A. Pain patients: traits and treatment. New York: Academic Press, 1974.

————. Psychological aspects of chronic pain. *Clin. Orthop.* 129: 150–55, November-December 1977.

Stone, C.I., et al. Coping with pain: a component analysis of Lamaze and cognitive-behavior procedures. *J. Psychosom. Res.* 21(6): 451–56, 1977.

Stone, I. Cancer therapy in the light of the natural history of ascorbic acid. *J. Int. Acad. Metabology*, vol. 3:1, 56–61, 1974.

————. Humans, the mammalian mutants. *Am. Lab.* 6:4, 32–39, 1974.

————. Hypoascorbemia, our most widespread disease. *National Health Federation Bulletin,* vol. 18, no. 10, November 1972.

————. Hypoascorbemia, the genetic disease causing the human requirement for exogenous ascorbic acid. *Perspectives in Biology and Medicine,* vol. 10, no. 1: 133–34, 1966.

————. Megascorbic therapy of the disease called leukemia. *Cancer Control J.,* vol. 2, no. 1: 1–4, 1974.

————. On the genetic etiology of scurvy. *Acta Genet. Med. Gemellol.* 15: 345–50, 1966.

————. Studies of a mammalian enzyme system for produc-evolutionary evidence on man. *Am. J. Phys. Anthro.* 23: 83–86, 1965.

————. The CSS syndrome, a medical paradox. *Northwest Acad. Prev. Med.* 1: no. 1: 24–28, 1977.

————. The genetic disease, hypoascorbemia: a fresh approach to an ancient disease and some of its medical implications. *Acta Genet. Med. Gemellol.* 16: 52–62, 1967.

————. The importance of fully correcting the genetic liver-enzyme disease, hypoascorbemia, in preventive medicine. In *New dynamics of preventive medicine,* ed. L. R. Pomeroy. New York: Stratton Intercontinental Book Corporation, 1974.

————. The natural history of ascorbic acid in the evolution of the mammals and primates and its significance for present day man. *J. Orthomolecular Psychiatry* 1:2, 3: 82–89, 1972.

Symposium on impressions of pain: a nursing diagnosis. *Nurs. Clin. North Am.* 12(4): 609–11, December 1977.

Symposium on pain (guest edited by J. Bonica). *Arch. of Surgery:* 112(6) pp. 749–88; 112(7) pp. 861–902.

Szasz, T.S. *Pain and pleasure; a study of bodily feelings.* New York: Basic Books Inc., 1975.

Szent-Gyorgyi, A. *Bioelectronics.* New York: Academic Press, 1968.

————. *Bioenergetics.* New York: Academic Press, 1957.

————. How new understandings about the biological functions of ascorbic acid may profoundly affect our lives. *Executive Health* 14(8), May 1978.

————. On oxidation, fermentation, vitamins, health and disease. Baltimore: Williams, 1939.

Taylor, C.W. Creativity: progress and potential. (Research conference on creativity held at University of Utah, June 1961.) New York: McGraw-Hill, 1964.

Ten minutes for everyone (editorial). *Lancet* 1 (8007): 344, February 12, 1977.

BIBLIOGRAPHY

Terenius, L. Significance of endorphins in endogenous antinocip-ception. *Adv. Biochem. Psychopharmacol.* 18: 321–32, 1978.
Thomas, L. *The lives of a cell.* New York: Bantam Books, 1975.
————. The future place of science in the art of healing. *J. Med. Education* 51, 23, 1976.
Tubesing, D.A. The wholistic health center project: an action-research model for providing preventive, whole-person health care at a primary level. *Med. Care* 15(3): 217–27, March 1977.
————. *Wholistic health: a whole person approach to primary health care.* New York: Human Sciences Press, 1979.
Turner, J.; Gallimore, R.; and Fox, C. *Placebo: an annotated bibliography.* Los Angeles: The Neuropsychiatric Institute, University of California, 1964.
Ubell, Earl. Health behavior change: a political model. *Prevent. Med.* I(1–2): 209–21, March 1972.
Usden, E., et al. Enkephalen: physiological implications. In *Neuroregulators and psychiatric disorders.* New York: Oxford University Press, 1976, pp. 319–28.
Victor, R., et al. Effects of biofeedback and voluntary control procedures on heart rate and perception of pain during the cold pressor test. *Psychosom. Med.* 40(3): 216–26, May 1978.
von Graffenrild, B., et al. The influence of anxiety and pain sensi-tivity on experimental pain in man. *Pain* 4(3): 253–63, February 1978.
Walker, J.M., et al. An analog of enkephalins having prolonged opiate like effects in vivo. *Science* 196 (4285): 85–87, April 1, 1977.
Wall, P.D. The gate control of pain mechanisms: a re-examination and re-statement. *Brain* 101(1): 1–18, March 1978.
Ware, J.E., Jr., and Snyder, M.K. Dimensions of patient attitudes regarding doctors and medical care services. *Med. Care* 13: 669–82, 1975.
Watson, G. *Nutrition and your mind.* New York: Harper and Row, 1972.
Weisenberg, M. Pain and pain control. *Psycho. Bull.* 84(5): 1008–44, September 1977.
Wepman, B.J. Psychological components of pain perception. *Dent. Clin. North Am.* 22(1): 101–13, January 1978.
Werner, A., et al. Teaching medical students interactional skills. *NEJM,* Special Article, May 30, 1974, p. 1232.
White, E.B., and White, K.S. *A subtreasury of American humor.* New York: Capricorn Books, 1962.
Whitehorn, J.C. Psychiatric implications of the "placebo effect." *Am. J. Psychiatry:* 114, 1958, p. 662.

White House conference on food, nutrition and health: final report. Washington, D.C.: Government Printing Office, 1969.

Whole person health care: an idea in evolution. Hinsdale, Illinois: Society for Wholistic Medicine, 1976.

Williams, R.J. *Nutrition against disease.* New York: Bantam, 1973.

Wolf, S. Effects of placebo administration and occurrence of toxic reactions. *JAMA:*155, 1974, p. 339.

———. The pharmacology of placebos. *Pharmacol. Rev.* II, 1959, p. 698.

Wolff, H.G. *Stress and disease.* Revised and edited by S. Wolf and H. Goodell. Springfield, Illinois: Charles C. Thomas, 1968.

# ABOUT THE AUTHOR

———

Norman Cousins is senior lecturer at the School of Medicine, University of California at Los Angeles, and consulting editor of *Man & Medicine*, published at the College of Physicians and Surgeons, Columbia University.

For almost all of his professional life, Norman Cousins has been affiliated with *Saturday Review*. He became its editor in 1940, a position he held for more than thirty years. He is presently its editorial chairman.

Mr. Cousins is the author of eleven books, including *Dr. Schweitzer of Lambarene*, *The Celebration of Life*, *Present Tense*, *In Place of Folly*, *The Good Inheritance*, and *Modern Man Is Obsolete*.